Work and the Mental Health Crisis in Britain

Work and the Mental Health Crisis in Britain

Carl Walker and Ben Fincham

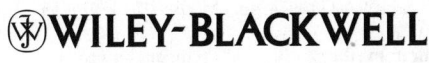

A John Wiley & Sons, Ltd., Publication

2011 © John Wiley & Sons, Ltd.

Wiley-Blackwell is an imprint of John Wiley & Sons, formed by the merger of Wiley's global Scientific, Technical and Medical business with Blackwell Publishing.

Registered Office
John Wiley & Sons Ltd, The Atrium, Southern Gate, Chichester, West Sussex, PO19 8SQ, UK

Editorial Offices
The Atrium, Southern Gate, Chichester, West Sussex, PO19 8SQ, UK
350 Main Street, Malden, MA 02148-5020, USA
9600 Garsington Road, Oxford, OX4 2DQ, UK

For details of our global editorial offices, for customer services, and for information about how to apply for permission to reuse the copyright material in this book please see our website at www.wiley.com/wiley-blackwell.

The right of Carl Walker and Ben Fincham to be identified as the authors of this work has been asserted in accordance with the UK Copyright, Designs and Patents Act 1988.

All rights reserved. No part of this publication may be reproduced, stored in a retrieval system, or transmitted, in any form or by any means, electronic, mechanical, photocopying, recording or otherwise, except as permitted by the UK Copyright, Designs and Patents Act 1988, without the prior permission of the publisher.

Wiley also publishes its books in a variety of electronic formats. Some content that appears in print may not be available in electronic books.

Designations used by companies to distinguish their products are often claimed as trademarks. All brand names and product names used in this book are trade names, service marks, trademarks or registered trademarks of their respective owners. The publisher is not associated with any product or vendor mentioned in this book. This publication is designed to provide accurate and authoritative information in regard to the subject matter covered. It is sold on the understanding that the publisher is not engaged in rendering professional services. If professional advice or other expert assistance is required, the services of a competent professional should be sought.

Library of Congress Cataloging-in-Publication Data

Walker, Carl, 1975-
  Work and the mental health crisis in Britain / Carl Walker and Ben Fincham.
     p. cm.
  Includes bibliographical references and index.
  ISBN 978-0-470-69977-5 (cloth)
 1. People with mental disabilities–Employment–Great Britain. 2. Work–Psychological aspects. 3. People with mental disabilities–Care–Great Britain. 4. People with mental disabilities–Rehabilitation–Great Britain. I. Fincham, Benjamin. II. Title.
  RC570.5.G7W35 2011
  362.196'8900941–dc22

                                                                                          2011006424

A catalogue record for this book is available from the British Library.

This book is published in the following electronic formats: ePDFs 9781119974239; Wiley Online Library 9781119974260; ePub 9781119974246; eMobi 9781119974253

Set in 10.5 on 13 pt Minion by Toppan Best-set Premedia Limited
Printed and bound in Malaysia by Vivar Printing Sdn Bhd

1   2011

Dedication

To Bree and our children Nancy and Joshua (Ben)

To Ruth and Anna (Carl)

Contents

About the Contributors	ix
Acknowledgements	xi
Chapter 1 Introduction: Mental Health, Emotional Well-Being and 21st Century Work	1
Chapter 2 Getting Britain Back to Work: A Policy Perspective	11
Chapter 3 Mental Health and Work-Experiences of Work *Ben Fincham, Carl Walker with Holly Easlick*	39
Chapter 4 Techniques of Identity Governance and Resistance: Formulating the Neoliberal Worker *Carl Walker, Ben Fincham with Josh Cameron*	67
Chapter 5 Managing Mental Health in Organizations	97
Chapter 6 Work/Life Balance and the Individualized Responsibility of the Neoliberal Worker	133
Chapter 7 Concluding Thoughts: Neoliberalism and the Shrine of Work	147
References	163
Index	179

About the Contributors

Carl Walker is a Senior Lecturer in the School of Applied Social Sciences, University of Brighton. His research and teaching interests include social inequality and mental distress, cultural representations of mental health, and critical community approaches to psychology. He is course leader for the MA in Community Psychology and is currently engaged in work around employment, personal debt and mental distress. His previous publications include *Depression and Globalisation* (2007).

Ben Fincham is a Lecturer in Sociology at the University of Sussex. He has been involved with developing projects on 'mobilities' and qualitative approaches to studying work in unstable employment environments, and his current research focuses on the complex relationship between work and mental health. He is co-author of *Mobile Methodologies* (2010).

Josh Cameron is a Senior Lecturer in Occupational Therapy in the School of Health Professions, University of Brighton. His teaching and research interests include: vocational rehabilitation; acute and community mental health care; occupational dimensions of resilience; and collaborative research. He has developed and leads a MSc module on *Vocational interventions for people with mental health problems*.

Holly Easlick is a postgraduate student from the University of Brighton. She has been involved with several research projects on mental health and psychosocial studies, and currently focuses on general health and well-being issues as a Health Trainer within the Portsmouth area.

Acknowledgements

First thanks to all the participants who gave their time to us and offered such honest answers to our questions. Thanks are due to Wiley-Blackwell publishers, particularly Karen Shield, for their valuable assistance in the development of this project. Thanks to Brighton University School of Applied Social Science for resourcing Carl through a sabbatical when much of his contribution to the work was completed (Carl would like to point out, despite the ordering of names on the cover, work was distributed evenly between the authors). Thanks must also go to the Community University Partnership Programme based at Brighton University especially Dave Woolf for part financing the research. Thanks also to colleagues at the University of Brighton and the University of Sussex, in particular Jayne Raisborough, Katherine Johnson, Mark Bhatti, Ruth Woodfield, Alix Brodie, Sally Jones, Becky Farmer, Anne Sheldrick, Karen Richards and Matt Adams. Particular thanks to Mark Erickson for his conceptual and theoretical guidance – any ideas you don't particularly take to are directly attributable to him. Special mention to Josh Cameron and Holly Easlick for their work on the project. Finally thanks to our partners, Ruth and Bree, for ideas, discussion and support during the production of this book.

Chapter 1

Introduction: Mental Health, Emotional Well-Being and 21st Century Work

> *It is very often the case that those who talk of the importance of the 'human factor' in one breath tell us that 'the main problem is attitudes' in the next. On the view taken here attitudes are no more suspended in mid-air than is technology . . . and 'attitudes' nearly always take us back to management. (Nichols, 1997: p. 117)*

There is a long standing interest in the relationship between mental health and work. However in recent years a consensus has developed both in academia and policy formulation that the number of people who are out of work as a result of mental ill-health constitutes a 'crisis' of public health care. Approximately one million recipients of incapacity benefit result from poor mental health and this represents 40% of the total people on incapacity benefit. Moreover this figure has increased from 26% in 1996 and will continue to be supplemented by an estimated 200 000 people with mental health conditions moving on to incapacity benefit each year (Black, 2008). The number of people currently on incapacity benefit has been constituted by Dame Carol Black as a serious failure of both employment support for the workless and of healthcare in the UK (Black, 2008). This has led to prominent calls for a desperate need for growth in publicly-funded mental health services in the UK (Layard, 2005). Indeed the sheer volume and variety of UK government policy documents in recent years that have been formulated to address the problems of those out of work with mental ill-health stands as testament to the postulated severity of this problem.

Work and the Mental Health Crisis in Britain, First Edition. C. Walker and B. Fincham.
© 2011 John Wiley & Sons, Ltd. Published 2011 by John Wiley & Sons, Ltd.

This 'crisis' sits against a backdrop of many studies that have highlighted the beneficial impacts of employment, counterpoised with the negative implications of joblessness (Bartley, 1994; Beale and Nethercott, 1985; Cohen, 2008; Huxley 2001; Lelliott and Tulloch, 2008; Rife, 2001; Zabkiewicz and Schmidt, 2009). As Huxley explains, mental well-being appears to be particularly sensitive to socio-economic influences (Huxley, 2001: p. 368). The obvious correspondence between high social capital and employment status is a determinant factor in feelings of self worth, and often alleviates stresses provoked by financial or employment insecurity. Alternatively the effects of joblessness and precarious employment are documented as impacting negatively on feelings of mental well-being (Gallie *et al.*, 1993; Hutchison, 2005; Karsten and Moser, 2009; Masterkaasa, 1996). This relatively unproblematic assumption of employment having positive effects and not being in work as having negative effects is made increasingly complex by the characterization of the labour market as changing – where precarious and non-standard employment are becoming the everyday reality of millions of people's experience of work and employment. The effects of working in such environments are reported to be complex, but for some sectors of the population working in casual employment has a detrimental effect on 'psychological well-being' (Bardasi and Francesconi, 2000). Using interviews with people from public, voluntary and private sector industries and with people who are attempting to enter or re-enter the job market having suffered mental health difficulties, this book examines the relationship between mental health and work in twenty-first century Britain.

The centrality of work to our lives clearly marks it out as influential in both the personal and socio-cultural realms and is one that is often uncritically referred to. Through policy and practices, the way in which work is organized and the ways in which we, as workers, are managed are key to understanding the reported levels of unhappiness and dissatisfaction that many experience at work. Long working hours, job insecurity or expectations of discontinuous employment, rather than being seen as anomalous to normal working lives, are becoming culturally instilled as 'the way it is.' There is research documenting the demoralizing effect of the increasing flexibilization and intensification of work, and a concern for this book is to garner a close perspective on what such changes mean to people. How are people making sense of their day-to-day work? How are people with mental health problems expected to integrate into situations that many are reporting as being bad for their health? How are those tasked with managing today's workers managed or expected to behave?

There is a considerable literature documenting the detrimental effects of long working days, job insecurity and, more generally, the potentially debilitating effects of work and employment in the twenty-first century (Gorz, 1999; Humbert and Lewis, 2008; Wang *et al.*, 2008). The severity of the problem is highlighted in National Institute for Health and Clinical Excellence estimates, where the number of work days lost due to illness amounts to 13 million a year at an estimated cost to the British economy of £28 billon (National Institute for Health and Clinical Excellence, 2009). At any one time 16% of working age adults in the UK are considered to have a mental illness, of whom up to half are seriously incapacitated, and when we consider that the current annual growth rate for mental health problems is in the region of 5%, then we can see that this is, if not a crisis, then certainly an area of grave concern for sufferers, employers and the government. As will be further illustrated in later chapters, the economic crisis of 2008 has further intensified the perception of a precarious employment environment where anxiety and depression are commonplace (Helm, 2009; Meltzer *et al.*, 2009).

Situated Perceptions and Work 'Cultures'

A concern for this book is not to deny the debilitating experiences of many workers in the UK, but to illustrate the role that particular cultures of work or perceptions of the experience of work contribute to a 'crisis' of mental well-being at work.

For many people their 'understandings' of their own health, often through the interpretation of health professionals, lead them into positions of mental ill health of varying severity. An initial visit to a GP can have profound repercussions for a person who has sought a consultation for the treatment of 'depression' or 'stress.' As Healy in particular has noted, the indiscriminate prescribing of SSRI (Selective Serotonin Reuptake Inhibitor) antidepressants can have serious negative consequences for a patient (Healy, 2006). The sorts of diagnoses and treatments offered are dependent on all sorts of factors – the confidence that a health professional (commonly a GP) has in a particular diagnoses, the predisposition the health professional has for particular types of treatment, what treatments are available in a particular area, the presentation of the person at the initial consultation and so on.

For those who suffer as a result of their jobs, the assessment of their psychological distress or damage will determine much of their subsequent engagement with work and the labour market. The psychological damage done at work will provoke a series of mechanisms that places them deep into mental health services, and state provided 'support' networks. For others, however, their engagement with support services will involve a trip to their GP, perhaps a limited amount of time signed off work, perhaps some antidepressants and an unsupported return to work. It is clear that consultations with GPs and others are important in establishing a route into mental health services or state-provided 'support' networks. As we have said, this is not to suggest that people are not suffering varying degrees of difficulty or distress, or that health professionals are behaving in a routinely improper manner. However, as we shall illustrate throughout the book, the position that people occupy in relation to discourses of mental health and work, in particular the positions in which they are placed by others – including health professionals, employers, colleagues, family and others – are key to understanding why it is that work and mental health have become synonymous with an interesting, and rarely addressed, dichotomy. That is, 'work' is good for people who are suffering mental ill health, and that many of those who are not suffering mental ill health report that 'work' is bad for them or makes them unhappy.

In data presented in this book the complexity in the relationship between mental health and work becomes evident. For those that have pre-existing or first episode mental health problems that are not considered to be directly caused by work there are particular issues for maintaining an employable persona. As will be discussed, the capacity of employers and colleagues to react supportively to others' problems is often mediated by the extent to which they are felt to have 'legitimate' reason to require support. This raises particular issues of disclosure to colleagues and also the judgemental, normalizing discourse of the deserving and undeserving 'sick' – that is to say who deserves support and who does not. As we illustrate, those whose problems stem from outside of work are often introduced into work places with attendant suppositions and subsequent behaviours towards them. The initial 'sick role' is often enforced by strategies and practices commonplace in places of employment – and levels of support are compromised by the economic or productive imperative.

Government Responses to Increasing Awareness of Mental Health Illnesses at Work

As we will discuss, with the cost of absenteeism spiralling, successive British governments have more recently attempted to introduce legislation and promote initiatives designed to support employers and employees with mental health related issues. It is interesting to note that whilst government has long been concerned with the impact of long working hours on certain parts of the workforce, an explicit engagement with mental health is relatively recent (Wainwright and Calnan, 2002: p. 3).

Two centuries ago policies started to emerge that recognized the need for conditions of work to be centrally regulated, and bound up in this regulation was the obvious recognition that people had to feel well to work. For example the 1802 Factories Act sought to regulate the working day, particularly for child workers, to between 8 and 12 hours. It also instructed factory owners to adequately ventilate their factories and attend to the outbreak of any infectious diseases inside their properties. However subsequent Factories Acts concentrated on the physical well-being of workers and almost no attention was paid to the mental impact of Victorian employment conditions. Throughout the nineteenth and twentieth centuries the spectre of work-related mental health problems appears to have grown unchecked. Wainwright and Calnan suggest that it really was not until the 1990s that the UK government Health and Safety Executive (HSE) began to take a meaningful interest in the issue of, in particular, work stress. That said the implementation of the Health and Safety at Work Act in 1974, and subsequent amendments, outlined responsibilities of employers to their employees' health as well as indicating levels of reasonable responsibility for employee health and wellbeing (HSE, 1974). Once again though, the *implied* concern with mental well-being in the Health and Safety at Work Act was not felt by some to be adequate for addressing the problem. In 1993 the Principle Medical Officer at the Department of Health wrote an article in *Occupational Medicine* entitled 'Mental health at work – why is it so under-researched?' In it he outlined the economic costs of mental ill health and, importantly, drew a distinction between 'stress' – and all of its attendant meanings, and what he referred to as 'clinical notions of health and illness' (Jenkins, 1993: p. 65). What the article indicated was that there was little empirical evidence from which policy could be derived. Jenkins called for 'accurate epidemiological prevalence studies' and 'research into techniques for primary, secondary and tertiary prevention' (Jenkins, 1993: p. 67).

Having drawn attention to the detrimental affects of depression, anxiety and other conditions Jenkins went on to co-author a relatively influential document 'Stress at Work: A Guide for Employers' (HSE, 1995). It has been argued that this was the culmination of an explicit engagement with the issue of mental health in the 1990s (Wainwright and Calnan, 2002: p. 3), and perhaps this is true, but the concentration on 'stress' has, we will argue, left many people marginalized through discourses of well-being and health at work. Whilst the guidance in the booklet was not compulsory it provided employers and employees with an indication of the symptoms and consequences of stress at work. However, there is an implicit assumption that the work and the well-being of the employee are solely causally linked. As has been suggested, this marginalized, and continues to marginalize, those with long standing mental health problems and also those whose problems cannot be easily ascribed to stress.

Work/Life Balance and Organized Support

Today there is a clearer understanding that there is a relationship between work and mental health that is worthy of attention. There is a psychiatric, psychological and more recently sociological concentration on the impact of work and employment on mental well-being. This more enlightened approach to work and health has lead to a number of strategies by policy makers and also activity in the voluntary and informal sectors. Supported employment schemes like the one used in one of our interview cohorts are becoming gradually more widespread, and the development of the concept of work/life balance have helped to make explicit the idea that there is a strong relationship between mental health and work and employment. However, another concern of this book is the extent to which strategies of support are appropriate to certain sections of the workforce. Once again it appears to us that some people who have been signed off work for a period of time, for instance with 'stress', and have not been referred elsewhere from an initial GP consultation and that such people fall between support networks that may be useful to them. The dichotomy of work and mental health – good for people that are unwell, bad for people that are well – is problematic for the contradictory positions of those who do suffer from mental health problems at work are placed. As will be illustrated, for those with pre-existing mental health problems the perception of the workplace as somewhere inaccessible to them is a cause of distress and discrimination – the levels and types of support required to shoehorn people into jobs in themselves serve to separate employees, as either easy and productive, or difficult and unproductive. On the other hand, those people who are not put into the systems of state or health institutional support are made responsible for their mental well-being in isolation, or with the occasional intervention of a GP.

We will illustrate an apparent individualizing effect through rhetoric of the work/life balance that is detrimental to people's feelings of well-being. By placing the onus of well-being at work as a balance with home life the responsibility of any employer for the mental health of their employees is diminished – in this discourse the key to happiness resides with employees getting the balance right.

Complimentary Perspectives of Mental Health at Work

The way in which mental health at work is framed can be examined from a number of complimentary perspectives. We contend that the relationship between mental health and work is framed in particular ways to serve particular ends, but that each perspective impacts on the experience we have of working, and our view of ourselves as healthy and productive workers. As we have already mentioned, the first is the governmental rhetoric that promotes the idea of work/life balance and flexibility. In this construct the onus of responsibility for one's mental well-being is individualized. An interpretation of this rhetoric is that work is accepted as being necessarily bad for people and seen as needing a positive counterweight – the 'life' part of a 'work/life balance'. An employer perspective on the mental well-being of employees is always mediated by the need to be fully staffed and economically 'productive'. As we shall illustrate, in this rhetoric the responsibility of the employer has to be tempered by economic considerations. Employee perspectives can be characterized as largely unsympathetic to those perceived to be emotionally needy thus provoking a judgemental discourse – that of being 'on the sick'. Whilst there are clear differences in terms of a hierarchy of power between government/policy maker, employer and employee positions in the labour market the three discourses outlined above do not exist in competition. They are supportive of a particular view of work as something that is to be coped with. If a person cannot cope then they have organized their work/life balance poorly. As well-being at work is an individual's responsibility employers can mobilize an economic or productive argument against employing or supporting workers in distress. Colleagues or co-workers frequently judge others who are getting into difficulty, or requiring support, as a sign of weakness or a source of resentment.

Clearly these observations are generalized and workplaces do not operate or react in such a linear or simplistic manner. However, our encounters with workers, with and without diagnosed mental health problems, have led us to conclude that these discourses are operating as regulators of 'reasonable' reactions to the issue of a relationship between mental health and the everyday experience of work.

Changing Labour Markets and Understandings of Mental Well-Being at Work

Whilst we would argue that the relationship between being at work and not being at work have never been as strongly demarcated in the past as is often implied (Fincham, 2008: p. 619), there have clearly been changes in the organization of labour in the UK that have had profound influences on the way we think of ourselves as workers. The increase of flexible labour (Bramham, 2006: p. 385; Taylor, 2001) and the perception of insecurity fuels a culture of long working hours and an excessive emotional investment in jobs (Gorz, 1999). Capitalist concerns with competing in a global labour economy, and in particular the assumption that the UK is increasingly a 'knowledge economy,' contributes to uncertainty and insecurity being a fundamental 'reality' of the organization of modern labour.

In *Reclaiming Work* Gorz illustrates the relationship between the micro and the macro. In his somewhat apocalyptic portrayal of the contemporary relationship between workers, their work and crucially their employers Gorz describes the process of 'subjection' where workers are inextricably allied to their corporate employers. With no particular affiliation to trades unions or class, people in current labour markets are made to feel grateful for being able to sell their labour and it is through this gratitude, Gorz suggests, that much exploitation arises (Gorz, 1999: p. 37–39, 52–53). It is clear from our data that people often work long hours and do more than their contracts imply because they fear that there is somebody waiting to give more to the job and ready to take the job if they do not prove their worth to employers. Global changes in trajectories of work and employment are having direct, mundane, everyday consequences for individual workers in the UK. Whilst this might be an obvious statement, it is often forgotten particularly when it is the individual that is being made to feel responsible for their happiness at work. A key point of this book is to support the idea that mental well-being and happiness at work are relational – the sorts of things that are happening at a governmental level are having direct consequences for our lived experiences of [and at] work.

The day to day experience of work for millions of people at work is defined by discourses of the direction of work and employment in the twenty-first century. Underpinning much of this book is the largely ignored relationship between the micro everyday experience of work and the macro organization of the global labour market – 'work' is popularly described as increasingly 'insecure' or unstable and psychological well-being is characterized by psychological stability and security. We argue, however, that this relationship – and importantly its particular discursive components – and how it is managed, has antecedents in the organization of labour at local, national and international levels.

Disciplining of Labour

The level of emotional and mental disquiet communicated by participants in this study has indicated a broader historical shift in the regulation of work and workers. As new technologies and strategies for flexible working have increased so the techniques for regulation and control have had to change. In the past labour has been disciplined through the requirement to be physically present, and 'hard' work was represented by the idea of arduous physical labour and its effects on the body. It is now disciplined by coping with pressure and intense mental or emotional activity. Of course in the UK this has accompanied the decline in manufacturing industries and agricultural work, but labour still needs disciplining and normalizing. Those that fall outside of this disciplining or normalizing regime are configured as difficult workers – and it is undoubtedly the case that those with mental health problems fall into this category. Throughout the book we will illustrate the point that behaviours that do not fit a 'normal' pattern of working or productivity are problematic to managers, who themselves are attempting to cope with regimes of discipline from their own managers.

There has been a perceptual shift to the realm of the psychological. In this shift those whose capacity to be mentally or psychologically productive increasingly find themselves victims of the increasingly intense and unhappy processes of twenty-first century work.

Organization of this Book

This book is organized into five further chapters. Chapter 2 examines in more detail the policy context within which our considerations sit. There is a recent historical overview of UK government attempts to keep everybody working, and discussion of developments in strategies in health promotion, flexible working and other policy initiatives aimed at addressing happiness and well-being at work or reintroducing people to work. Chapter 3 presents data from interviews with employees and managers from across the private, voluntary and public sectors. The data is organized into themes, rather than sectors being dealt with discretely. This is because we have found that, whilst there are clearly differences in terms and conditions between the three sectors, many of the key issues that have arisen in terms of mental well-being are common to all. Using data from interviews, chapter 4 addresses the experiences of those that are attempting to retain or re-enter the job market whilst suffering a diagnosed mental illness. Chapter 5 examines the contribution of occupational culture to considerations of mental well-being and happiness at work and chapter 6 examines inherent contradictions in the way that discourses of work/life balance are mobilized in UK workplaces. An extended conclusion in chapter 7, contextualizes the previous material through a consideration of the problematic 'dialogue' between psychology and labour. The book finishes with comments and recommendations for practice.

Chapter 2

Getting Britain Back to Work: A Policy Perspective

As has been pointed out in the introduction to this book, recent figures on days lost to mental ill health and the subsequent impact on the economy present a bleak picture. The movement in recent years in the UK from manufacturing to a more poorly paid service sector-oriented employment profile is only expected to continue to compound this problem since service sector employment is associated with a higher prevalence of stress-related illnesses. This chapter has two purposes. The first half provides an overview of the dominant academic and policy logics assembled in recent years to combat what has generally been constituted as a growing problem of mental health and work. The second half provides a critical appraisal of these ways of knowing and directing the conduct of people whose mental health has proved problematic to their work narratives. This critique locates these dominant logics within broader modes of social, political, economic and discursive organization in recent years.

There has been a considerable body of recent academic work to extol the virtues of work on well-being. In an independent review commissioned by the Department for Work and Pensions. Waddell and Burton (2006) examined the scientific evidence of the health benefits of work and found a strong evidence base generally showing that work was good, and indeed therapeutic, for physical and mental health and well-being. Drawing on Jahoda's theoretical framework on the psychosocial functions of work, Goodwin and Kennedy (2005) found that work was beneficial because it facilitated a structure to the day, self-confidence and social contact in a way that not working generally did not. There is also literature on the mental health benefits of employment that suggests that these benefits are not confined to adults who work. A report in 1982 by Valliant and Valliant of 456 inner city males who were prospectively followed from 14 to 47 years of age suggested that the capacity to work in childhood predicted the employment success of underprivileged participants in adult life (Vaillant and Vaillant, 1982). Indeed this capacity for paediatric toil was considered to be more important than social class and all other childhood variables in predicting adult mental health and the capacity for interpersonal relationships.

One expected corollary of the axiomatic construction of work as central to subjective well-being is the notion that unemployment is generally not a good thing. Unemployment has major implications for households and the causal link between unemployment, quality of life and poor physical and mental health has by now been well established (Gallie, et al., 1993; Masterkaasa, 1996; Hutchison; 2005). Moreover there has been a plentiful source of empirical research in recent years that has documented not only how beneficial work is for the healthy functional worker, but how beneficial it can be for those experiencing mental ill-health. For instance, we know that depressed people who work are healthier than their non-depressed counterparts (Elinson, et al., 2004). We also know that an enjoyment of work can have a positive influence on a person's mental strength (Irvine, 2008), and that being away from the work context can lead to social isolation, and often profound financial hardship. Indeed, a report from the Secretary of State for Work and Pensions (2002), noted that such forms of often brutal hardship are not the only problematic association between employment and mental health. Not only are the pernicious effects of unemployment a genuine social challenge but the acceptance of these circumstances as permanent, of developing an 'unemployable identity,' means that such people become harder to help (Secretary of State for Work and Pensions, 2002). This is of particular significance because the retention of employment, even unpaid employment, has an apparently profound effect on more life domains than any other medical or social intervention (Huxley, 2001).

Contrary to popular public perception, the majority of mental health service users want to work. For example a study in 1996 by Seebohm and Secker showed that of 77 day centre clients interviewed, 61% said that they wanted help to return to work (Seebohm and Secker, 2005). The same authors noted that, on the whole, 95.7% of mental health service users would take some form of paid employment be it full, part-time or self-employed, and that 69% desired further education or training. However for people who have been on incapacity benefit for a prolonged period the outlook as regards their opportunities to work is far from optimistic. From the 1996 Labour Force Survey, Huxley (2001) reported that 85% of people with long-term mental illness were not working. Of those who have only recently made the switch to incapacity benefit, the prognosis is equally bleak. After 6 months on incapacity benefit it is thought that people had a 50% chance of returning to work, a figure that diminishes to 25% after 12 months. After two years on incapacity benefit only 10% of mental health service users are recorded as having returned to work (Rinaldi and Perkins, 2005).

It seems clear that absence from work through the context of mental ill-health constitutes a serious problem to a number of stakeholders in the UK. As one might expect, at the forefront are the experiences of the people who are struggling with their mental health. The suggestion that these people are growing in number is a deeply worrying trend that is played out in different ways for those who are responsible for the often daily struggle of concomitantly managing their work commitments and mental health identities. This could be someone who is continuing to struggle at work despite being seriously unwell, it could be someone who has been absent from their work premises for a prolonged period as they seek to address their mental health difficulties prior to returning to work. It may include people whose mental health difficulties mean that they find it difficult to work continuously without using small periods of sick leave during the time when their suffering feels incommensurate with performing adequately in work. Whatever the work context, it is clear that there are a growing number of people whose mental health problems make it difficult for them to attend work in what one might cautiously term a standard manner. This in turn could be problematic for two other key stakeholders. As outlined in the introduction it could be problematic for employers who stand to directly lose money as a result of productivity loss and/or absenteeism. Moreover it is a clear problem for the Exchequer who lose substantial and increasing sums of money in the form of reduced tax revenues and increased payment of incapacity payments.

Systematic and strategic interventions to move people from incapacity benefit back into work are not novel but the deliberations of recent years have been formulated through the construction of simplistic dichotomies that fail to capture the complex and contradictory cultural, political and social influences at the heart of employment and mental health. The credibility and integrity of many incapacity benefit claimants has been central to the identities of the major political parties in the UK. A right of centre agenda, and its associated rhetoric, has a considerable and proud history of representing such claimants as pernicious and malingering drains on public resources. The discursive muscle of the traditional UK right has frequently been mobilized to construct incapacity claimants as barely credible miscreants whose lack of personal responsibility and eagerness to exploit the tax payer requires tough political action. The Left has traditionally resisted such pervasive suspicions of mistrust and welfare abuse, instead displaying a tendency to construct incapacity claimants within a recovery discourse where people are viewed as sites for disability management, specialist rehabilitation and support. However the inception of New Labour and 'compassionate conservatism' has prompted a perceived reformulation of the traditional political orientations of the major UK political parties in recent years with a corresponding clamour by Right and Left to present themselves as the true denizens of the centre ground. These political reconstructions, together with the substantial and growing body of evidence suggesting that work is beneficial for both our mental and physical health, have provided the context for successive administrations to make employment central to their management of mental health.

UK Government Policy on Employment and Mental Health

Concern regarding the costs of incapacity benefit has been a key element behind recent UK government policy that has been forceful in its representation of the central importance of employment to mental well-being. Drawing on discursive constructions of both work-as-therapy and work-as-human-right, there was a proliferation of documentation that outlined the New Labour government's intention to facilitate work in the lives of the workless. The policy interventions and delivery guidelines have been broadly based around two central conceits. Firstly, there is the need to provide a helping hand to mental health service users who are currently failing to engage with the therapeutic benefits of the workplace. That is, there is a need to get more people with mental health difficulties into work. As such, there has been a significant attempt to facilitate individual interventions that will contribute both to the reduction of stress in the workplace and to the treatment of those with mental health difficulties such that they are made ready for the workplace. These interventions are intended to address the mental health needs of those identified as having difficulties and will ameliorate their symptoms such that they are able to retain or indeed gain work. The second strand of policy formulation is predicated on the need to establish healthy working environments in order to remove one of the risk factors that can potentially contribute to the deterioration of an employees' mental health and to an inhibition in the process of recovery.

In 2006 the Department of Work and Pensions outlined details of their 'New Deal for Welfare' which outlined the importance of these policy strands. This document stated that enabling citizens to enter the world of work had been a guiding principle of the government's drive to create a modern active welfare state since 1997 (Department of Work and Pensions, 2006). Moreover, they proposed to create healthy workplaces and improve access to good quality occupational health. This vision for employment, mental health and well-being has been supported by other recent government publications (HM Government, 2005; Department of Health, 2007) that have included a concerted focus on improving mental health literacy in organizations and an increase in productivity.

Getting People into Work: The Interventions

In recent years the message that work is central to addressing the difficulties of mental health service users has been promoted through a number of public sector and government publications (HM Government, 2007). The National Health Service Mental Health National Service Frameworks (National Health Service, 1999) sought to spell out national standards for mental health, what such standards should achieve, and how such achievements could be realized. The document noted that unemployed people were twice as likely to have depression as those in employment and so employment opportunities and training were posited as central to the bettering of people's lives within a health context. The Office of the Deputy Prime Minister (2004), reiterated the Department of Work and Pensions' target to increase the employment rate of people with disabilities and stipulated that everyone with a mental health problem should have access to an employment advisor.

Increasing frustration at the significant increase in incapacity benefit claimants in recent years, combined with the fact that 40% of those claiming incapacity benefit will not make the transition to work, has fuelled a desire to develop new ways of understanding the problem of UK incapacity benefit (The Secretary of State for Work and Pensions, 2002). A pragmatic philosophy that combined early ongoing support, direct access to a comprehensive range of provision, and clear financial incentives to move people back to work came to represent a multifaceted solution. One of the key initiatives to address these needs in recent years has been the 'Pathways to Work' programme. Pathways to Work utilizes a number of incentives and interventions in order move the focus from what people cannot do to what they can do. Work-focused interviews, where new incapacity benefit customers meet with personal advisors to discuss their work ambitions, and a tax-free return to work credit providing security for the change, have been formalized in order to provide the necessary financial and occupational support.

However, qualitative research carried out recently on the Pathways to Work programme suggested mixed results (Hudson, *et al.*, 2009) both on its compatibility with NHS treatment and on the satisfaction of clients, some of whom felt pressurized to apply for job vacancies that they felt were unsuitable. Moreover the jobs that clients entered tended to be low skilled and concentrated in the service sector. A report on the European Social fund (Third Sector European Network, 2006) also criticized Pathways to Work for its tendency to target people closer to the workforce.

While Pathways to Work focuses on the financial and work-oriented barriers to employment for people with mental health difficulties, further policy has focused on interventions to treat people who are experiencing poor mental health and has been based on a seemingly robust literature that has sought to provide evidence for the efficacy of individual treatment solutions both inside and outside of the workplace (Byrne, 2005; Brouwers *et al.*, 2006).

The focus of solutions to the problematic nature of mental health and work that have emerged from the evidence base of the mainstream psychological and psychiatric sciences in recent years have ranged from relatively holistic and sometimes platitudinous lifestyle interventions to those with a greater therapeutic focus. Firmly situated in the former camp, Byrne (2005) lamented that, while excessive work stress can be traced to excessive workload, bullying, continual change and a lack of challenge, some of the key ways to combat this stress include eating regular and healthy meals, exercising regularly, managing your time well, learning breathing exercises and 'counting your blessings at the end of each day'. Dorio (2004) stated that the relatively low average job tenure in a supported employment programme (70 days) suggests that perhaps a more holistic alternative be utilized to meet employer and employee needs. The author presented a social and vocational rehabilitation programme called the 'Clubhouse model' as a potential solution. This model emphasizes positive attitude, setting realistic goals, having an open mind and seeing beyond the moment as central to prolonged employment success.

On the more formally therapeutic side of the evidence base a number of variants on the central tenets of Cognitive Behavioural Therapy (CBT) have been posited as the most efficacious ways in which to address the difficulties associated with mental health and employment. A recent paper in the Netherlands evaluated the cost effectiveness of an intervention based on CBT for a group of people whose 'minor mental disorders had led to sickness absence'. This protocol was found not only to increase motivation but was also well received by both patients and professionals (Brouwers et al., 2006). The general ethos of such approaches is supported by Schneider et al.'s, (2002) call for an individualized model of rehabilitation to promote the right conditions for success in work. This is based on their key finding that poor social skills hinder people who struggle with mental health problems and employment and that, as above, positive attitudes to work are crucial in helping service users to get and keep jobs.

Few studies have attempted to formulate and/or compare organization-focused interventions with those focused on the actions, beliefs and emotions of the individual. Van der Klink and colleagues (2001) undertook a meta-analysis which compared CBT relaxation techniques, multimodal programmes and organization-focused interventions. They found that although stress management was effective, CBT was maximally effective; that is, more so than any other type of intervention although it should be noted that very little detail was provided on the nature of the organizational interventions and at what level(s) they operated. Of 48 studies only 5 focused at the organizational level and the authors suggest that it may be that it takes longer for the effects of such interventions to be realized at the individual level. In highlighting the beneficial and practical impacts of a range of stress management techniques, Seymour and Grove (2005) stated that limited evidence was found to suggest that a focus on organizations rather than individuals produced superior results in reducing people's mental health problems. Indeed they stated that individual rather than organizational approaches to managing common mental health problems were most likely to be effective and that for those with common mental health problems at work the most effective approach was cognitive behavioural in nature. Partially supporting this, Gardner and colleagues (2005) showed that, for work-related stress, participants in the cognitive therapy groups showed a significant improvement at follow-up. Those in the behavioural group showed a smaller but still clinically effective improvement.

The majority of recent work on cognitive and behavioural interventions have used CBT, and there is a substantial and growing body of work that has presented cognitive behavioural therapy and closely related treatment programmes, as optimal or recommended interventions for employee well-being, reducing work-related stress and improving work outcomes (Della-Posta and Drummond, 2006; Lysaker *et al.*, 2009; Millward *et al.*, 2005; Palmer and Gyllensten, 2008; Park *et al.*, 2004; Proudfoot *et al.*, 2009; Ruward *et al.*, 2007). Indeed work that fails to highlight significant and/or optimal benefits for the cognitive behavioural family of interventions is indeed a rare beast (De Vente *et al.*, 2008). However the emergence of CBT in the employment field should not be taken as evidence of its unilateral efficacy at addressing the problems mentioned. In evaluating a job retention service intended to support GPs in preventing unemployment among patients with mental health problems, Thomas *et al.* (2005) found that vocational counselling aimed at planning a return to work, anxiety management, assertiveness and confidence building was found to be useful.

Before the latter sections of this chapter offer a critique of the theoretical assumptions that underpin much of this work it is important to draw links between some of this key evidence and the continuing development of UK policy in the field of mental health and employment. Work related stress, work productivity and the task of transferring incapacity benefit claimants with histories of poor mental health into work have very much come to be recognized as a problem, or series of problems, that require individual solutions. These solutions are aimed primarily at ameliorating, supporting and resilience-building with the 'sick' individual. Indeed much of the evidence base above represents a collective of ideologically congruent interventions that are predicated on the basic notion that the optimal locus for solving work related mental health issues is that of the person who is suffering.

Toward the end of New Labour's first term in office, the picture for mental health funding in the UK was relatively bleak. The share of mental health funding in NHS and social service budgets was falling and the progress of delivering the government's reform agenda was considered to be patchy and uneven around the country (Sainsbury Centre for Mental Health, 2003). However, in 2005 the prominent economist Richard Layard wrote an influential report that explicitly located a rapid return to work as an outcome for mental health services and articulated a desperate need for a growth in publicly funded mental health services in the UK (Layard, 2005). Indeed Layard called for an extra 10 000 therapists and 5000 clinical psychologists to be trained in the coming five years. The answer to Layard's call, and to the growing concern over the cost to the economy of the increasing number of people with mental health problems on the incapacity benefit register, was the development and proliferation of the Increasing Access to Psychological Therapies (IAPT) programme.

The NHS IAPT programme has one principal aim and that is to support primary care trusts in implementing National Institute for Clinical Excellence (NICE) guidelines for people suffering from depression and anxiety (National Health Service, 2008a). That is, to essentially utilize the results of the evidence base above to bring about effective treatment for people with depression and anxiety. World Mental Health day in 2007 saw Health Secretary, Alan Johnson, announce a three-year funding package designed to allow 34 primary care trusts to implement IAPT services such that more than 900 000 people in the UK would have access to treatment. The plan was for half of this number to move to recovery and hence reduce the number of people on incapacity benefits. Indeed this was and is a key metric of the IAPT programme. As well as seeking improvements in the mental health of the people who use the programme services, IAPT is being evaluated on its ability to deliver people with mental health difficulties into employment. The key performance indicators of IAPT are reducing the number of people on sick pay and benefits, improved patient experience and the facilitation of social inclusion (National Health Service, 2008b). While there is variance in the way that IAPT is realized in different geographical areas, the key services used to deliver these targets are CBT, both computerized and interpersonal, signposting and bibliotherapy (reading relevant self-help material).

An initial assessment of IAPT certainly appears promising. Up to this point the achievements included 5500 people referred during the 13 months covered by the report. Although the scale of follow-up was clearly relatively short, at the end of the treatment 5% more of the treated population were in some form of employment and both sites achieved a recovery of 52% for people with depression and/or anxiety (Clark, 2008).

Healthy Workplaces

The Health and Safety management standards

Thus far, there has been an outline of the institutionalized strategy of presenting work as a target for those struggling with mental health problems, a strategy that has been actioned through a focus on the individual as the unit of treatment and principally through cognitive behavioural interventions. Indeed the IAPT scheme was largely predicated on this very set of assumptions. We also know that Seymour and Grove (2005) and Van der Klink *et al.* (2001) hold little faith in the relative efficacy of workplace or organizational changes as the locus of action in the battle to address the difficult relationship between mental health difficulties and prolonged employment. However, in recent years the UK government have stated on a number of occasions that reforming the practices and organization of UK workplaces is also paramount to ensure work environments that are not toxic to the mental health of workers. There is an often-stated desire to provide work environments that are welcoming, accepting and accommodating for those who are suffering with a mental health problem or returning to work following prolonged sickness absence (HM Government, 2005; National Health Service, 1999; The Secretaries of State for the Department of Work and Pensions and the Department of Health, 2009a).

Coffey and Dugdill (2006) note that the UK government have explicitly set out to promote health at work by improving working conditions and central to this trajectory is the UK Health and Safety Executive Management Standards Approach (The Health and Safety Executive, 2005). These standards were developed specifically to reduce work-related stress in British workers and cover six key areas of work design that include demands at work, control or consultation with workers on work patterns, relationships at work and employee support. The Health and Safety Executive have made it clear that employers have a duty to ensure that risks arising from work activity are properly controlled and that systems should be in place to respond to individual concerns, including concerns over bullying. It states that 'The leaflet contains notes on good practice which are not compulsory but which you may find helpful in considering what you need to do' (The Health and Safety Executive, 2005). The guide for employees in the same document suggests that employees 'should speak up if you are experiencing a problem, and talk to your manager to find a win-win situation' (The

Health and Safety Executive, 2005). In an employment utopia where relations between employer and employee are characterized by open lines of communication, mutual respect and a common purpose such advice would undoubtedly prove perfectly pragmatic. This combination of information for employees and guidance for employers is considered by the Health and Safety Executive to be sufficient in order that 'the new standards mean managers will now have to work with you to find solutions, so your problems should reduce over time' (The Health and Safety Executive, 2005). Such optimism suggests that the Health and Safety Executive are possibly unfamiliar with some of the institutionalized modes of discrimination and marginalization experienced by many workers with mental health problems (outlined in further detail below). In a government document of the same year called 'Health, work and well-being- Caring for our future' (HM Government, 2005), it was articulated that the HSE was working with organizations across the public sector to deal with the growing cause of sickness through stress by adopting this management standards approach. This was the primary strategy to address the 256 000 new cases of workplace ill health in 2003/2004 that resulted from stress.

Exactly what these management standards mean to employers and employees will be revisited in later chapters as part of the empirical work carried out in the South East of England. For now, however, it is sufficient to point out some clear potential issues. One of the key problems is that HSE guidance is not legally binding (Robinson and Smallman, 2006) and on average companies can expect a visit from HSE inspectors approximately once every 17 years (Wainwright and Calnan, 2002). Likewise, Taylor *et al.* (2003) list the HSE items under good practices that are not enforceable and, as such, rely on managerial prerogative. They found that, in reality, at least as far as call centres were concerned, managers are more likely to take action to remedy problems with the physical environment than to address elements of the generic organization of work that might impinge on sickness absence. Indeed with the endemic decline in union representation there is little organized resistance that might ensure that employers comply with HSE regulations (Robinson and Smallman, 2006).

The Black Report

In 2008, Dame Carol Black undertook a government review (Black, 2008) in order to identify the factors that stand in the way of good health and to elicit strong interventions and services in order to overcome these factors. As mentioned earlier it started from the supposition that the sheer numbers of people currently on incapacity benefit represented a serious failure of both employment support for the workless and of healthcare in the UK. She noted that the current approach assumed that sickness was incompatible with work. Black brought workplace setting and structure to the centre of the debate by suggesting that there needed to be a shift in attitudes such that both employers and employees know the role of the workplace in promoting both health and well-being. One of the impediments that currently provided a degree of inertia was the fact that many employers were characterized as still being unsure of the strength of the business case for implementing workplace initiatives that promoted health and well-being. Line managers were positioned centrally in the process of identifying, supporting employees and maintaining regular contact with employees who were off work in a sensitive manner. Black proposed a new 'Fit for Work' service based on a case-managed multidisciplinary approach addressing people's treatment and advice needs in the early stages of sickness absence. A case manager would refer into a wide range of services that might include traditional NHS services as well as less traditional but relevant advice services specific to the client's practical needs. Following this service recommendation it was decided that various Fit for Work models would be tested (Secretary of State for Department of Work and Pensions, 2008) and evaluated, and that these projects may well link with IAPT initiatives around the country.

The 'Fit for work' pilots were scheduled to run until at least 2011. They are expected to reduce the time that service users take to return to sustained work and reduce the number of people losing employment and moving into incapacity benefit as a result of ill health and, particularly, poor mental health (HM Government, 2009). The programmes are proposed to involve such interventions as skills advice, employment advice and liaison, including conciliation to overcome disputes, as well as psychological therapies including, as mentioned earlier, possibly linking with IAPT therapy services. The focus of this programme, unlike IAPT, is not solely based around the provision of NICE-approved psychological therapy or self-help in order to move people back into work. The 'Fit for work' schemes also have an arm that opens up the possibility of addressing some of the social and relational problems that may arise from mental health at work and subsequent sickness absence, including potential conflicts and tensions.

Following the Black report, the Secretaries of State for the Department of Work and Pensions and the Department of Health (2009a, 2009b) published the first national framework for mental health and employment where the broad ethos was to improve health and well-being at work for the whole population. More specifically this framework seeks to ensure that managers use the HSE competency framework for line managers and encourage employers to commit to training for managers to support mental health and well-being. As such, it appears clear that the focus of intervention at the line manager level is based around knowledge production. There is also the intention to encourage employers to train managers in absence management, rehabilitation and job retention. The key aims of the framework however are threefold. Firstly, there is the intention to challenge mental health stigma and prevailing cultures of low expectations around mental health service users. Secondly, they intend to mobilize preventative interventions at the individual level by teaching skills that support resilience and well-being in schools and through other services. Finally, they outline a desire to promote the five steps for mental health and well-being. These are connecting with people, being active, being curious, learning and giving. Examples of how these five steps are realized include such advice as going for a walk or cycle, noticing the changing seasons, savouring the moment and doing something nice for a friend or stranger (Secretaries of State for the Department of Work and Pensions and the Department of Health, 2009b).

Up to this point this chapter has attempted to provide an uncritical appraisal and brief outline of recent UK employment and mental health policy up to the present. The principal and enduring themes that characterize not only government policy but a great majority of academic consensus in the field are as follows. Firstly, work, generally speaking, is good for people's mental health and, as such, people who are experiencing mental health problems should be, wherever possible, encouraged to stay in work (if they are employed) and start work (if they are not employed). By and large there is little deviation from this theme. Now of course mental health itself is a difficult concept to pin down. In reality it represents an enormous and varied series of personal experiences and rich tapestries of suffering, incapacity, wellness, ability and competencies. However, broadly speaking, whatever your type of suffering, and however it has been caused, work will be better for you than not working.

Secondly, when people do experience mental health problems, and particularly what are referred to as 'common mental health problems', depression and anxiety, they tend to be better treated at the individual level and CBT appears to be the most effective way to do this. As such we have the mobilization of the IAPT programme. With the possible potential exception of some Fit for Work pilots, interventions that focus on work organization and cultures, or the social relations of work, tend to be relatively marginalized.

Thirdly, healthy workplaces are a good thing and a key facilitator for individual physical and mental health and HSE management standards have been developed to ensure that employers are aware of the health implications of such prominent contours of the occupational arena as control and demands at work, work relationships, support at work and consultation through change. However the degree to which employers pay attention to these HSE management standards depends very much on the caprice of the individual employer since adherence to these standards is essentially optional.

To reiterate much of this approach to work and mental health, Perkins, Farmer and Litchfield (2009), in a review commissioned by the Secretary for Work and Pensions, reiterated that employment actively improves mental health and well-being. Indeed it recommended that employment outcomes for people with a mental health condition form part of the key performance indicators and commissioning criteria for Department of Work and Pensions, Health and Social Services. The review recommended that employment specialists should be embedded in primary care and secondary mental health teams.

In order to consider possible perspectives from which to critique the various activities above, the following sections will explore some of the key theoretical and empirical work that frames the way that neoliberal economic policy has proscribed changes to the ways in which people are expected to enact, manage, negotiate and indeed recover into work identities in the UK.

A Critical Appraisal of Changing Employment Landscapes

Since the end of the 1970s there has been a substantial consensus regarding the notion that the UK political and economic landscape has been characterized by a neoliberal economic regime positing free market economics as the solution to social needs (Gorz, 1999; Gray, 1998; Stiglitz, 2002; Walker,

2007). In order to stimulate economic regeneration following a series of political and economic crises in the 1970s, corporate interests were placed at the heart of the political agenda. Indeed the UK has not been alone in adhering to the tenets of this right-of-centre focus on the supply side of the economy.

> In country upon country, markets were deregulated, state planning and power dismantled, welfare was cut and/or criminalized and full employment policies abandoned. Low tax, privatization and the demonization of government regulation were celebrated as panaceas for a declining social order. (Walker, 2009: p. 67)

However, while this essentially monetarist approach to managing the economy had and has its supporters, any evaluation that judges it by social or egalitarian criteria that focuses on the quality of people's lives makes it very difficult not to conclude that the institutionalized changes of the last thirty years have been largely responsible for inflating both social inequality and the number of people in the UK living in poverty (Gorz, 1999; Gray, 1998; Walker, 2007).

Recent years have seen no reduction in the trend toward greater inequality and economic disparity and by 2002 the richest 1% of the UK owned 23% of the country's wealth (it was 18% in 1986) during a period when the country's wealth has increased (Williams, 2006). Moreover in the late 1990s the distribution of personal wealth has continued to grow more unequal and in 2001, in a table of national income inequality, Britain came fourth in the European Union (Williams, 2006). Perhaps unsurprisingly this economic climate has led to lamentable figures on poverty and child well-being. A recent UNICEF report (UNICEF, 2007a) showed that children in the UK were among the worst off in Europe with UK children ranked twenty-first out of twenty-five EU countries in a number of indices of child well-being. The scale of relative poverty in the UK is particularly problematic with nearly 13 million people and nearly 30% (3.8 million) of children living in relative poverty. This figure is considerably higher than the majority of the United Kingdom's European neighbours (Luxembourg Income Study, 2009; Walker, 2007) and the UK has the fourth worst income poverty of twenty-four OECD countries (UNICEF, 2007b). Of particular consequence is the statistic that no OECD country devoting 10% or more of GDP to social transfers has a child poverty rate higher than 10%. Likewise no country devoting less than 5% of GDP has a child poverty rate of less than 15%. The UK rate is around 30% (UNICEF, 2007b). In recent years we have experienced a 'credit bubble' driven by consumer and national debt that arose as a result of Western economies searching abroad for cheaper production bases (Turner, 2008). Turner (2008) suggests that weak financial institutions, regulatory authorities and political firmaments, in thrall to the Anglo-American business model, have led to an economic climate where debt rises remorselessly and bad financial practices drive out good.

In the UK, house repossessions, redundancies and over-indebtedness have soared as a result of the credit crunch. The number of house repossessions in the UK jumped by 48% in the first half of 2008, the highest for 12 years, and unemployment in the UK rose by 131 000 between September and November 2008, the highest since September 1977. As of October 2009, 25% of people in the UK were currently struggling to cope with their monthly bills and 39% described themselves as 'being in trouble' if they had to find £50 extra per month (Creditaction, 2009). Furthermore, the fact that 64% of people on annual incomes of less than £9,500 have problem debt suggests that the experience of personal debt is particularly distressing for those living in relative poverty (Department of Trade and Industry, 2005). If we reject the Malthusian celebration of the beneficial equalizing properties of capitalism, then we are left with the inescapable conclusion that there exists a political and economic climate that has specific and often pernicious effects on our social environments. Nowhere is this better illustrated than with the context of work. Any understanding of employment and mental health must sit against this backdrop of economic and political market liberalization.

In recent years we have witnessed the successful reification of 'Globalization' as the somewhat disingenuous 'global spread of science and technology'. However, in practice this has been little more than a branding exercise, albeit an effective and pervasive one, that essentially masks the movement of neoliberal economic ideology from the few to the many. In a nuanced and eloquent neo-Marxist exposition of labour markets in the age of globalization, Andre Gorz (1999) noted that recent systems of employment have restored the worst forms of domination, subjugation and exploitation, not to mention a gradually diminishing stock of available work. According to Gorz, a historically unprecedented mass of capital is producing ever-growing volumes of wealth production while consuming less and less labour. The need for European companies to achieve US profit rates and provide regular and substantial shareholder dividends has led to a series of circumstances that can be characterized as capital reaffirming its status as the sole possessor of sovereignty. This means effectively having the power to control taxes as a result of inclining nation states to compete against each other to attract capital (Navarro *et al.*, 2008; Genschel *et al.*, 2002; Bauman, 1998a). On the subjective level of individual workers, Gorz contends that no physical or psychical space remains that is not occupied by company logic. Rarely has the domination of the conditions and price of labour by business been quite so acute and this is evidenced by the fact that in Britain 95% of new jobs are either part-time or fixed-contract (Gorz, 1997). This set of social and economic conditions has created an unusual paradox in that we are being urged to desire work in permanent jobs since this constitutes not only the means with which to live in relative comfort but access to an acceptable social identity. However this very same work is disappearing fast.

A central feature of the chain of events that has led to Gorz's employment dystopia has been the institutionalized deunionization of the UK workforce. Indeed, since the 1980s, the reduction in union power has meant that the consequences of work re-organization and intensification have been less likely to be contested (Taylor *et al.*, 2003). Union presence at UK workforces fell from 73% in 1980 to 54% in 1998 (Millward *et al.*, 2000), and Wainwright and Calnan (2002) contend that this erosion of workplace solidarity and collective power has been central to the development of the work stress discourse as a central, if desperate, tactic of employee empowerment in today's labour markets. This contention is critically appraised in greater detail in the context of our own data in chapter four.

The combination of theory and conjecture above will remain at the level of speculation without an attempt to contextualize it in the lived experiences of the people working in the UK today. There is a growing body of research on these lived experiences that proves instructive and tacitly provides an evidence base for some of Gorz's broader contentions on the changing dynamics of Western employment. According to Purcell and colleagues (1999) employers appear to be increasingly using various forms of numerical, functional and pay flexibility in order to maximize labour force productivity at the lowest labour costs. This has meant an increased probability of being in fixed-term or temporary employment, increased staff hours worked and a wider range of working responsibilities (Hudson, 2002). The commendation that Gordon Brown received from the International Monetary Fund in 2007 regarding the UK's refusal to implement robust labour protection has been embodied in employers' execution of modes of labour flexibility that are not currently available to many of our European partners (Jenkins, 2007).

In 1998 the Job Insecurity and Work Intensification study (JIWIS) of twenty UK workplaces (Burchell *et al.*, 2002), a series of communications with senior managers, line managers and employees, found that the modes of flexibility outlined by Purcell *et al.*, (1999) were a result of dominant stakeholder pressure which then results in an increased intensity and duration of work (Lapido and Wilkinson, 2002). These changing patterns of flexibility have meant that households, and particularly women, are less able to exercise control over their economic and social situations today than have been in the recent past (Hyman *et al.*, 2005). Indeed in some cases, in the software industry for instance, management have had discretion to vary start and finish times by up to two hours with 48 hours notice, a situation compounded by pervasive cultural expectations of unpaid overtime (Hyman *et al.*, 2005). Cully and colleagues (2000) have noted that fixed term and zero hour contracts have grown over the past decade and report that about 3/5 of workplaces used both contractors and one other form of non-standard labour.

According to Robinson and Smallman (2006) it is these specific flexible employment practices that have some of the most marked associations with injury and illness. Although Burchell (2002) found little evidence for any overall change in job security in recent years, they did find evidence for rising work stress levels as a result of increased work intensification from the 1980s through to the end of the 1990s. Indeed in a 1999 UK survey of the members of the institute of management 70% of respondents experienced an increase in workload in the previous 12 months. Further, the UK stands out amongst other countries in Europe as regards this increase in work intensification. This finding was echoed by the European Foundation for the Improvement of Living and Working Conditions (2000) whose report on ten years of working conditions in the EU, which included 21 500 workers across the member states, found that work is becoming increasingly intensive with over 50% of workers now working at high speed or to tight deadlines for at least a quarter of their working time. The modes of flexibility discussed above were widespread and temporary work remained a strong employment characteristic with 10% of employees on fixed-term contracts.

The changes outlined above have profoundly influenced the way that many people respond to their working environment, not least the institutionalization of corporate cultures that are increasingly defined by performance orientation (Cunha, 2001). Wichert (2002) used the JIWIS data to show that, under certain circumstances, being employed can be more stressful than being unemployed. The data suggest a strong relationship between this increase in work intensification and three outcome measures including psychological outcome using the General Health Questionnaire. Indeed work intensification has an even stronger negative psychological outcome than job insecurity. The HSE (2005) stated that 1 in 5 people currently find work stressful and that over 500 000 people reported experiencing work-related stress at a level that they believe made them ill. Moreover there was a 15% drop (from 35%) in the proportion of men completely or very satisfied with the number of hours they worked, 22% for women (from 51%) (Taylor, 2000). In UK call centres Taylor et al. (2003) reported that more than 2/3 of workers felt quite or very pressurized as a result of work on a 'normal' day and that 74% of call handlers believed that targets contributed either a great deal or to some extent to feeling pressurized.

For those whose changing work environments do not allow a space to remain at work while experiencing mental health difficulties or, indeed, directly contribute to mental health difficulties, there is often very little strategic policy in many organizations to address these mental health needs. In a postal survey of workplaces in Sefton, Merseyside in 2001 (Coffey and Dugdill, 2006) it was agreed that there had been an increase in flexible employment practices and work intensification and that these are the primary causes of health problems. However while 2/3 of workplaces felt that they needed advice on ensuring the health of their workers and 51% of workplaces identified a stress management policy as one they would like to produce, the perceived barriers to developing policies included lack of time/money (70%) and not having the expertise (37%).

It should be noted that whilst many academics in the field accept that institutionalized changes in UK work cultures have been characterized by a greater degree of work intensity, employer flexibility and work stress, the literature is not unanimous. While Taylor agrees that the proportion of flexible working hours rose from 16.8% in 1992 to 22% eight years later, and that this change was significant, he does not generally concur with the notion that there is any evidence of a 'new' kind of employment relations that could be characterized by the 'end of the career' (Taylor, 2000). He notes that 92% of workers still held permanent contracts. Sweet and Meiksins (2008) agree that there is undoubtedly evidence of longer hours and new forms of insecurity but they are more sceptical of any claims that this somehow represents tacit evidence for a new economy as much as simply reflecting the machinations of the old economy – that is, the continued effort of employees to find the least expensive ways to produce goods.

The Experience of Mental Health at Work

Contrary to the rhetoric of the UK tabloid press, there is little room for doubt in the literature regarding the majority of mental health service users' desire to work. However there is also little room to doubt that the experiences of mental health service users in work are complex, challenging and, at times, incredibly painful. Rinaldi and Perkins (2005) noted that the majority of those with serious mental health problems can gain and sustain employment so long as they are party to the right kind of support. However, the considerable body of research that outlines being in work as inherently better than not being in work should not automatically be read as work being good for mental health service users, especially when we factor in some of the institutionalized changes in the cultures of work in the UK in recent years. There is a considerable body of literature to suggest that mental health service users who work can very often experience extraordinarily difficult environments.

To understand the real extent of the complexity of the experiences of people at work it is important to draw on or to formulate work which allows an exploration of power, discourse and subjectivity. As the traditional mainstream psychological sciences research and attendant government policy discussed earlier shows, there is often an uncritical acceptance of corporations as naturally existing community entities (Deetz, 1992); entities whose practices and policies leave little space for, or inclination to, understand the nature of potentially egregious patterns of social relations that they can embody. As a result of this ideological acceptance of their natural and inevitable forms as constituted through the traditional drives toward productivity, many theorists have shown a greater inclination to explore issues of corporate and/or employee efficiency and effectiveness. However, a closer scrutiny of organizations reveals struggles of power and identity where complex, contradictory and shifting identities and subjectivities (Knights and Wilmott, 1989) relate to very distinct social practices. McKinlay and Starkey (1997) noted that organizations are social machines in that they produce elaborate discourses of information and knowledge and that such discourses frame the tactics of power that so many employees find themselves subject to. Miller and Rose (2008) outline the centrality of technologies of government, assemblages of persons, techniques and institutions for conducting conduct, for constituting and rendering knowable personhood in ways that compliment prevalent political rationalities. In the case of the post-industrial workplace satisfactory subjectivities take the form of self-regulating neoliberal agents whose capacity for deliberative choice allow them to cope individually with any work circumstances they encounter (Gill, 2008).

Moreover very rarely do we find that the identities and subjectivities enabled and marginalized within these specific neoliberal discourses exist free of negotiation and resistance. Rather they can be the site of regular and complex struggles (Clegg, 1997). These forms of identity negotiation are fundamental because once they become fixed they permit only certain ways of knowing the self and of knowing the organization lest employees find themselves subject to practices of social or procedural discipline. Line managers have a central role in these social practices and in the enablement, reproduction and policing of certain normative and acceptable employee identities. The inherent demands of productivity that so often fall on the shoulders of line managers ensure this. The demands of production outlined earlier often increasingly inhibit identities beyond that of worker and as and when such alternative identities do manifest themselves they are often reconstituted as deviant, divisive and problematic to both colleagues and management. In many cases the people who have transcended the acceptable boundaries of work identity are subject to subtle forms of domination (Deetz, 1997) and disciplinary power through stigma, resentment and processes of organizational discipline and estrangement that can lead to dismissal or voluntary employment severance on the part of the employee.

Seebohm and Secker (2005) stated that a number of their focus groups led them to the conclusion that the stigma of being mentally ill is a major barrier and that experiences of stigmatization had the effect of sapping peoples' confidence and motivation to work. Indeed one of the main barriers to employment included employer attitudes to the mentally ill, a feature noted by 83% of respondents. The WHO identified stigma related to mental health as the most important issue in the field and stated that unemployment rates for service users are between 80–90% (Stuart, 2004). Yet few people who attend community mental health teams in the UK get any kind of help to tackle the institutionalized stigma and discrimination that they face (Seebohm, 2005). 78% of mental health service users in Bristol reported having lost one or more jobs as a result of mental illness and between a third and a half were dismissed, were forced to resign or were made redundant due to discrimination (Thomas and Secker, 2005). This work is supported by Thornicroft (2006) who stated that 47% of mental health service users described experiences of often incredibly painful discrimination at work.

In a recent review for the Department of Work and Pensions, a descriptive piece of work found that supporting an employee with a mental health problem could place significant demands on the time of line managers (Sainsbury *et al.*, 2008), time that Gorz claims our increasingly productivity-oriented cultures of work simply do not allow. Perhaps unsurprisingly, few people with mental health experience were optimistic about what their employers were actually able or prepared to do for them to help and support them to work. Sainsbury and colleagues found a general openness among employers to take on employees with mental health conditions (Sainsbury *et al.* 2008), but then in the current climate of disability discrimination awareness, such a response might not be particularly surprising. Partially contradicting this work, Stuart (2004) found that in the US 33% of mental health service users had been turned down for a job which they were qualified for once their mental health problem was disclosed and that in the UK 58% of employers would never hire someone with depression for an executive role (and only 5% lower for a clerical position). Thornicroft (2006) reported that the mention of a mental illness significantly reduces the chance of getting a job.

Where problems have arisen, line managers often fail to prove adept at understanding and effectively managing these experiences. Irvine (2008) showed that workers with mental health difficulties had a range of experiences with employers but that responses to their difficulties tended to be based on individual attitudes rather than organizational approaches. Line managers often found it hard to understand the long-term and gradual nature of recovery. A lack of understanding by line managers was likely to impact on their responses to workers with mental health problems and may in part explain Nieuwenhuijsen *et al.'s* (2004) finding that supervisor behaviours is a predictor of the return to work of people on sick leave with mental health problems.

A number of the pieces of work on stigma and discrimination have tended to be descriptive in nature and so do not allow a comprehensive understanding of some of the social practices and processes that underpin the way that stigma and indeed mental health are performed in work contexts. In a nicely observed study of return to work practices, Eakin (2005) noted that an industry has grown around the return to work phenomenon including regulatory provisions, disability management, rehabilitation programmes, assessment tool production and professional training. Eakin highlights a prevalent discourse of abuse in the policy and practice of return to work and states that this discourse has pernicious effects on experiences of injured or ill workers. This discourse refers to pervasive and institutionally embedded expectations that participants in the work injury compensation and support system will abuse its entitlements. She found that workers often return to work prematurely in order to allay accusations of illegitimacy and described the phenomenon of injured and ill workers being required to 'perform' their personal credibility and integrity both to line managers and colleagues.

To draw this section together, the UK is currently experiencing an historic peak in the capacity of business to dominate the conditions and price of labour. As such, there has been a concomitant growth in experiences of work intensification and job insecurity (Burchell *et al.*, 2002; European Foundation for the improvement of living and working conditions, 2000). This has provided a fertile context not only for an increase in work-related stress and ill-health but for line managers to exhibit a reduced capacity to be able to manage the long-term and sometimes fluctuating needs of workers with mental health problems (Irvine, 2008). Alongside this there have been sustained and significant accounts of institutionalized stigma and discrimination in employment contexts.

However, despite these potential problems, UK government policy and academic consensus in the area of sickness incapacity generally, and often unproblematically, constructs work as a panacea for recovery from mental health difficulties (Clark *et al.*, 2008; Cohen, 2008; HM Government, 2005; Lelliott and Tulloch, 2008; The National Health Service *Mental Health National Service Frameworks*, 1999; Zabkiewicz and Schmidt, 2009). Moreover, as discussed above, person-focused interventions suggest that focusing on eating regular and healthy meals, exercising regularly, managing time well, learning breathing exercises, counting your blessings at the end of each day, doing something nice for a friend or stranger (The Secretaries of State for the Department of Work and Pensions and the Department of Health, 2009a), engendering positive attitudes to work, setting realistic goals and improving social skills are all key to the recovery process that allows people to resume work. Some of these personal changes, together with a number of others, have been formalized into cognitive behavioural therapy which has been considered to be the most effective tool for those with common mental health problems at work (Seymour and Grove, 2005).

Despite most health promotion focussing on individual aspects of employee health like health behaviours and medical conditions (Musich *et al.*, 2006), opinion is far from unanimous that individualized interventions are optimal for the broad structural, economic and social relational changes outlined above. Parslow and colleagues (2004) noted that, as a general rule, an individual's options for reducing work stress were far more limited than an organization's options, which might include better recognition of modification of tasks and management strategies. It is not only the qualities or capabilities, or indeed thought processes, of the individual worker that are paramount in the quality of experiences of mental health service users at work. Musich *et al.* (2006) found that increased presenteeism (health-related on the job work impairment) was significantly associated with poor working conditions, ineffective management/leadership and work/life imbalance and the authors stated that there was growing evidence that organizational aspects of work life, including job design, job efforts and rewards, could have a major impact on the health status of employees. The authors suggest that mainstream approaches to health promotion at work have been too narrow in focus. Deery *et al.* (2002) suggested that to understand emotional exhaustion, situational rather than person-centred factors are key. These include such factors as workload, role overload, work pressure, and role conflict. Indeed service sector employment, the big UK growth sector of recent years, is particularly characterized by work that is intensive, frequently stressful and repetitive; emotional exhaustion is commonly related to a management focus of quantity, routinization, and role overload.

Using the Labour Force Survey in England and Wales to better understand the rehabilitative processes for both ill and injured workers, James *et al.* (2006) found that organizational commitment and culture, including attitudes and values of both line management and senior management, were important. Moreover, there was a good deal of scope for encouraging employers to do far more for ill workers, possibly through legal requirements. For workers with mental health problems it was shown that support by the supervisor had an influence on the incidence of periods of short-term sickness absence. This is of particular significance since in 71% of organizations the supervisor was responsible for the return to work process

(Nieuwenhuijsen *et al.*, 2004). Some service users who left their jobs complained that their colleagues treated them differently once the mental health issues became clear. Moreover the qualities of the supervisor, such as their ability to communicate openly and provide a degree of fairness and support were key. Non-working service users mostly described a lack of support from their supervisors, and indeed increased stress due to their supervisors, as crucial elements in their negative experiences (Kirsh, 2000).

The importance of organizational climate is emphasized by Ylipaavalniemi *et al.* (2005) whose cross sectional evidence suggests that unfavourable team and organizational climates are associated with high stress. Indeed poor team climate (characterized by little worker involvement in decision making and unclear or unattainable objectives) is the strongest predictor of depression in workers regardless of age, sex and income. Further studies in recent years have supported the importance of relational aspects of work environments (Sveinsdottir *et al.*, 2006), management style and culture (Friesen *et al.*, 2001) and workplace bullying (Niedhammer *et al.*, 2006) in both the generation of occupational stress and success or failure to return to work.

Interestingly, the US workplace, is rather stronger in implicating the workplace and employer's prerogative as the principal source of the stressful workplace. Stefan (2002) suggested that the American workplace is permeated with 'an organizational perversity where abusers are often protected and the victims punished' (Stefan, 2002: p. 112), where there is currently a skewed and unhelpful acceptance that employees are viewed as having the problem. One might suggest from UK interventions into our workplace mental health experiences that we share a similar ideological bias. Perhaps Tony Blair's pride that Britain had the most lightly regulated labour market of any leading economy in the world Wainwright and Calnan (2002) may yet prove to be part of the problem rather than the solution to effective and healthy workplaces.

Concluding Remarks

The work in this section highlights evidence for the way that social relations and organizational cultures impact on workers' health. However this evidence is not visible to any notable extent in UK mental health and employment policy. So where does this work leave policy initiatives to treat individuals with a view to returning them to the therapeutic environs of the workplace? According to McGowan (2009), the National Institute for Health and Clinical Excellence for all its merits, simply fails to offer a system that can capture the range of broader interventions that address key social issues and that there is a tendency to produce 'unhelpfully limited answers to complex social problems' (McGowan, 2009: p. 467). This is a frustration that has been echoed by White (2008). Central to the 'Pathways to work' scheme and IAPT initiatives has been the positioning of mental health service users as requiring individual, largely context-free advice or therapy in order to allow them to benefit from the immeasurable and universal effects of being employed. The conversion of the UK to a workfare state has seen a transformation in the relations and identities that characterize employment and unemployment. Citizens are coerced, supported and pushed into assembling a particular therapeutic project of the self based around their capacity to work (McDonald and Marston, 2005). The dominance of the 'work as beneficial for psychological recovery' discourse positions the UK government as an intermediary between the universally favourable context of work and the isolated and individualized suffering of those with 'disorders'. The growth in problematic low-wage work, the continued reduction in the availability of permanent work, an increase in work intensity, a refusal to effectively legislate through the Health and Safety Executive on the workplace conditions, and the endemic marginalization and abuse of many people with mental distress (Eakin, 2005; Seebohm and Secker, 2005; Stuart, 2004; Thomas and Secker, 2005; Thornicroft, 2006) makes any such dominance problematic. As the research above illustrates, relational aspects of work are hugely influential in determining well-being. Individuals do not 'work' in isolation, rather they are involved in complex sets of relations with other individuals, institutions and working cultures. An understanding of the experience of being at work as political and relational undermines the rationale for an entirely individualized, and to some extent pathologicizing, approach to those experiencing difficulties at work. This perspective not only provides a challenge to the ethos of individualized intervention exemplified by the IAPT programme but it also represents a challenge to the ideology of much of the psychological academic research in the field.

The following chapters, and indeed the rationale for this book, are based on the contention that we simply do not know enough about the ways in which employer's and employees experience mental health at work in the UK. We would echo the call from Kirsch (2000) who states that gaps exist in the literature regarding the meaning and impact of work. The way the workplace impacts on people has largely been ignored in the quest to provide rationales that support the discursive construction of employees as an effective locus of intervention for problems that are often beyond employees' control or imagination. James *et al.* (2006) suggest that there is a weakness in the rehabilitative evidence base that is represented by having too few studies that look at the context of ongoing employment relationships. Most work in the field has consisted of quantitative surveys with little in-depth exploration of the organizational dynamics that surround the management of these processes. Moreover there has been a heavy reliance on studies from the USA, Australia and Scandinavia and too little work on small and medium-sized enterprizes (Coffey and Dugdill, 2006).

We know that the social relations of work are important and that line managers often struggle to manage the mental health of their employees. We also know that they interact in some way with current HSE guidelines. We know there is a wealth of experiences of stigma and discrimination and that a great many people are working in environments characterized by increasing labour intensity and work stress. However what we know less about is exactly how this complex matrix of social, economic and political relations interface with each other in the spaces where people try to manage both their mental health and the mental health of others. There is much to know if we are to effectively evaluate both government policy on work and the significant academic literature on the value of stress reduction and CBT. There is a lack of up to date, detailed work that explores the ways that mental health and work experiences are constructed, negotiated, constrained and at times, marginalized. The clamour to put people to work has left little space to explore the potential problems in doing so. The following chapters represent an attempt to do that.

Chapter 3

Mental Health and Work-Experiences of Work

Ben Fincham, Carl Walker, with Holly Easlick

Introduction

Key concerns for this book are work-experiences that might contribute to a sense of mental malaise, ill health or unhappiness. Previous research, particularly in occupational psychology (Gallie *et al.*, 2003; Goodwin and Kennedy, 2005; Hutchison, 2005; Waddell and Burton, 2006) highlights the importance of work to well-being. The purpose of this chapter is not necessarily to refute previous claims but to represent the concerns of people working at the beginning of the twenty-first century and to relate these concerns to our theoretical position on work and well-being. Our primary focus is on the idea of cultures of work as establishing the ground on which our understanding of acceptable practices and reactions to work are based. These cultural formations provide the social backdrop to our working selves and our experiences of work.

For us an important constituent component of contemporary cultures of work is people's perceptions of broader patterns in labour markets. This is to say that people do not understand their position as workers in isolation to other parts of the labour economy. As Doogan explains our understanding of work as insecure is in relation to understanding the labour market more generally as full of insecure jobs (Doogan, 2009: p. 201–2), this then becomes a self fulfilling prophesy as contracts become less favourable to employees on the premise that work is insecure. Accepted wisdoms

Work and the Mental Health Crisis in Britain, First Edition. C. Walker and B. Fincham.
© 2011 John Wiley & Sons, Ltd. Published 2011 by John Wiley & Sons, Ltd.

about contemporary work are products, as Doogan puts it 'manufactured' (Doogan, 2009: p. 194), designed for maximizing productivity and masquerading as culture. Whilst there is much written about 'new' configurations of work (see for example Castells, 2006; Hudson, 2007; Kalleberg, 2009; Sweet and Meiksins, 2008), we have drawn on older literature to enable our analysis of contemporary work and mental health. Baldamus, Illich and Gorz wrote about how to theoretically frame the experiences communicated to researchers of work, employment and health. Reading their work in a modern context illustrates two key points. The first is that the way we *experience* work has not changed radically over time – even if *forms* of work have. Second that there are existing theoretical orientations that, despite their age, have much to tell us about work, individualism and mental health. The purpose of outlining elements of the work of these three scholars is to place the narratives that we identify through the interviews into radical interpretations of our place in wider social and economic networks.

Baldamus wrote throughout the 1960s and has an enduring influence on studies of work and employment – even if it is rarely credited – to the present day (Erickson and Turner, 2010b: p. 8–9). It is his 1961 classic *Efficiency and Effort* that we find a particularly useful critical view of contemporary work and mental health. As opposed to the traditional view of industrial relations being most commonly understood as naturally harmonious and abnormally disrupted by conflict, Baldamus thought quite the opposite (Erickson, 2010: p. 36). His observation that industrial relations are 'a structure of differentiated power that reflects unequally distributed advantages and disadvantages' (Baldamus, 1961: p. 7) underlined the importance as he saw it of recognizing the inherent conflict of worlds of work. Erickson notes the key question for Baldamus:

> When we look in depth at what work actually involves for many, the meanings attached to work and the costs of work to the individual in terms of stress, workplace conflict, alienation and ill health, the real question we need to address isn't why people stop working, but why they work at all. (Erickson, 2010: p. 36–37)

For us the resonance of this way of looking at work is clear. Rather than examining what is going wrong for people at work which would normally be characterized as positively functional, this perspective suggests examining what is good for people in an environment that is normally negatively functional[1]. It is perhaps this observation that permits partial answers to the question 'Why is work thought of as good for people that are mentally unwell and bad for people that are mentally relatively healthy?' Baldamus' view allows for both a macro and micro analysis of experiences of work, in ways that were not particularly accessible at the time at which he was writing. Sociological considerations of work and employment have been characterized by an ongoing epistemological entrenchment – most simplistically expressed by preferences for particular methods – either quantitative or qualitative. Baldamus advocates a perspective on work that takes as its starting point data drawn from individuals and then places them in what we might now call a psychosocial framework led primarily by the observation that work will be experienced in conditions of disharmony. There is a clear relationship between the micro level individual data that may be gathered and its relative position to a macro assumption about the nature of work and in particular industrial relations. Whilst extrapolating from micro to macro level assertions is of course nothing new, in the field of work and employment the sorts of positions made possible by Baldamus' work in *Efficiency and Effort* are not well used. As an example, his analysis of 'work realities' involved a similar methodological position as the one adopted in this book – an examination of how people describe work rather than relying on common sense assumptions about what work involves or people's feelings towards it.

For Baldamus, experiences of *tasks* at work are more than the sum of their parts. Unhappiness often spreads to other areas of activity and to other aspects of occupation. In order to make clear these relationships Baldamus refers to the impacts of various 'realities' of work (Baldamus, 1961: p. 76). Jobs involve varying physical conditions, and involve varying amounts of repetitiveness and routine and these can be experienced as negative or positive depending on various contextual constraints and the relationship that these three conditions have with each other.

Throughout the analysis of the data gathered specifically for this book, but also in relation to other empirical studies cited here, it is worth bearing these interrelated aspects of doing a job in mind. Baldamus makes no claims about the inherent impacts of particular regimes. Repetitiveness can be experienced as either tedium or traction – and it is in the narratives from people at work that a sense of how people are experiencing work can

---

[1] This is illustrated most clearly later in the chapter in the sections 'Relationships and Perceptions of Others' and particularly 'Goal Orientation and Achievement'.

be found. Obviously Baldamus was writing in a very different labour environment than today, but as will be illustrated by our analysis his observations are still pertinent to understanding the position currently occupied by discourses of mental health and well-being and the individual worker in twenty-first century employment in the United Kingdom.

Where Baldamus offers an account of experiences, Ivan Illich begins to contextualise the individualised accounts that emerge from Baldamus. The aftermath of the financial turmoil in 2008–9 has provoked much discussion of appropriate responses to crises. Indeed the title of this book is *Work and the Mental Health Crisis in Britain*. For Illich the mobilization of this sort of language provokes legitimacy for particular societal responses that masquerade as being for the common good. At the beginning of his book *Toward a History of Needs* (1978) Illich provides a resonant précis of what 'crisis' indicates:

> *Crisis* has come to mean that moment when doctors, diplomats, bankers, and assorted social engineers take over and liberties are suspended. Like patients, nations go on the critical list . . . *Crisis*, understood in this way is always good for executives and commissars, especially those scavengers who live on the side effects of yesterday's growth: educators who live on society's alienation, doctors who prosper on the work and leisure that have destroyed health, politicians who thrive on the distribution of welfare which, in the first instance was financed by those assisted. (Illich, 1978: p. 4)

In Illich, there are accounts of the standardization of experience, the dominance of expertise and professionalism, and the obscuring of a sense of proportion through 'corrupted language' (Illich, 1978: p. 29). Important for our purposes is Illich's use of a concept of conviviality. It is in his critique of mechanization that our use of the concept lies – in a non-convivial workplace the function of the worker is simply to maintain the working of the system, or for Illich, the machine. This lack of conviviality stifles creativity and produces the sorts of environments that are ripe for exploitation by the professional elites that are described in *Toward a History of Needs* (1978), particularly in a piece entitled 'Useful Unemployment and Its Professional Enemies'. Illich describes work (and not being at work) as being dictated by a 'hegemony of imputed needs' (Illich, 1978: p. 29) where 'language, the most fundamental of commons, is . . . polluted by twisted strands of jargon, each under the control of another profession' (Illich, 1978: p. 29). In a discursive sense we understand this as particularly important when analyzing data from contemporary interviews. The deployment of particular language as enabling or disabling is evident, as will be illustrated[2].

This elaboration of the position spelt out in the earlier *Tools for Conviviality* (Illich, 1973) allow us to once again reflect on the perspectives on a changing labour market a generation ago. The startling thing for us is that, whilst the working environment might have changed, our reactions to such changes retain a logic that can be traced from Baldamus through Illich, and André Gorz.

In, *Reclaiming Work*, Gorz charts the decline of economic nationalism and the rise of post-fordism and all that the term entails. The break in Western Europe with mass production as the defining feature of competitiveness – this capacity is transferred to the ability to produce a variety of products in shorter times and the advent of 'lean production' – is key to understanding a modern relationship to work and importantly how particular assumptions about cultures of work have arisen. Whilst much of the latter part of *Reclaiming Work* sets down Gorz's agenda for a radical reorientation of work and productive labour, for us the most illuminating section lies in his account of contemporary labour relations. For Gorz a prominent feature of modern employment is to be found in what he calls 'subjection.' Implicit within 'lean' productive techniques is the idea that if team management and autonomous working decrease waste and increase efficiency, (however they are defined), to achieving a pre-prescribed objective then it should be encouraged or pursued – defined as post-Taylorism by Gorz. He then goes on to point out that the potential liberatory aspects of post-Taylorism – autonomy and freedom – could only materialize with the dissolution of capitalist social relations. However, workers tend to be employed in post-Taylorist settings in the UK when they have been stripped of their class identity and of their place in and membership of wider society – the very identities that protected against the debilitating effects of capitalist social relations (Gorz, 1999: p. 36). Cast free from these more traditional discourses of identity as a worker, employment relations take on a pre-modern formation where workers in particular workplaces are encouraged to think of themselves as part of a family, and the relationship between the company and the corporate work collective becomes the only social bond. An obvious implication for workers is that self-worth is gauged through a

---

[2] This point is discussed in more detail further in the chapter in the sections 'stress and anxiety' and 'perceptions of others'.

relationship with their employer or firm. If the firm does not want them the worker feels useless. According to Gorz 'the company bought first the person and their commitment and only then did it develop their capacity for abstract labour' (Gorz, 1997: p. 38). Contemporary capitalist social relations are predicated on the idea that workers consult and reflect and 'be the autonomous subjects of production' without realizing that this autonomy is already delimited by the company and will be directed to pre-ordained goals – in other words a mirage of autonomy.

Relationship to Cultures of Work

As we have explained we are not suggesting that there is necessarily anything new in these affective reactions to working situations, indeed quite the opposite. We draw on several key theorists in order to frame our argument: Experiences of contemporary work are part of the logic that stretches from increasing deindustrialization in the UK in the 1960s, through the latter half of the twentieth century to the present day. Much of this chapter is drawn from interviews conducted in 2008–09 at the beginning of a recession. These interviews are with men and women working across the private, public and voluntary sectors predominantly in the South East of England. These contemporary accounts are examined in the light of our understanding of a radical strain of older literature concerning work, individualism and culture that we believe is helpful to explaining individual responses to the global labour market – illustrated so devastatingly in the aftermath of the financial crisis of 2008–09.

With Baldamus' assertion that working relationships are not predicated on harmony – rather conflict – people experience disharmonious working environments where they are encouraged to think of themselves as in some way determining their circumstances and working relationships. It should be no surprise that so many people report work as being a place that is impacting negatively on their sense of identity, self or – to use a pathology – mental health.

With Baldamus, in the early 1960s, the human reactions to processes and cultures of work are to be found, with Illich in the 1970s the relationship to managerialism, standardization in the name of diversification, and the role of market intensity is illustrated, and moving into the late 1990s, Gorz's explanation of the transformation of work and individual responses to such changes – and to a certain extent bringing Baldamus and Illich together – are highlighted. Using these three theorists in particular, our orientation to work as operating at macro and micro levels simultaneously, structurally process bound and individually affective, temporally mutable and politically charged is explored.

Thematic Presentation of Data from Interviews

The themes are derived from the interview data and are presented as such but will be argued to be constituent parts of what people are identifying as contributing to their sense of well-being at work. These relate closely in a broadly structural sense to what we are calling 'cultures of work'. The themes we concentrate on are: time/hours of work; the role of technology in work; the relationships with others and the perception of others; anxiety/stress; and goal orientation or achievement. These emerged throughout the interviews as key concerns for people when asked to reflect on their feelings about their work. Interesting elements of the analysis of the data are the things that were not as prominent as we had originally assumed they might be. Of particular note are tiredness and fatigue, which were obliquely referred to in relation to long hours of work. Possibly respondents took it for granted that we would assume that they were tired if they were working long hours, or that the language for fatigue is couched in terms of stress or anxiety. Another element largely absent from the discussions was money, and reasons for these omissions from the interviews will be discussed later.

In terms of the organization of the themes in this chapter, as with the presentation of much qualitative data, the boundaries between the apparently discrete sections are blurred. There is a lot of overlapping and inter-relatedness of themes and we will draw attention to these crossovers throughout the discussion of the data and appropriate literature.

Time and Hours of Work

In almost all of the interviews across the sectors, and irrespective of position in a workplace hierarchy, the issue of time and time management was mentioned, and more often than not re-iterated at different points in the interview. Extended hours of work appear to be commonplace and the examples here are drawn from across sectors and employment positions. It appears that there is a widespread acceptance that many jobs cannot be properly performed within the hours of what one might call the traditional eight hour working day. The ways in which people tended to explain their working day was relatively straight-forward. There was broad acceptance that working long hours is a factor in modern employment in the UK. For example a Deputy Head Teacher spoke unproblematically about the length of her working day:

> I mean I stay to work until quite late anyway so I'm here to sort of 7, yeah between 6 and 7 unless there's a parents evening in which case it would be later, but between 6 and 7 most nights and I'm here at 7 in the morning. (Deputy Head Teacher)

She then went on to rationalize these extended hours, and her work at weekends as reasonable due to her not having children of her own. A Human Relations Consultant when describing work she had done with lawyers stated that there was:

> ... the expectation that you don't leave work 'til half past 7... Most of them you have to work to 10–11 at night. (Human Relations Consultant)

In the voluntary sector a worker in a mental health charity in south east of England attributed the extension of hours to the contraction in funding allied to a sustained expectation of service. The halving of a team with the same amount of work to do was clearly going to impact on the hours required to deliver various tasks. Another interviewee working in the public health sector spoke about the length of her working day:

> Being in at 8, getting in at 5 for the children and then starting work again at 8.30 and doing until about midnight, just to literally get things in order. (Public Sector Health Worker)

She then went on to describe the hours of her husband, who worked for a large American corporation as being '24 hours on call' (Public Sector Health Worker). The relationship between long working hours and culture is interesting. It has been reported as a feature of British work for many years (see for example Crewe, 1999; Demos, 1995; Jones 1991; Wallop 2009). In this sense long hours might be part of an acculturated feature of working in the UK – it is just what happens here. However long working hours might be a symptom of the wider systemic observations provoked by Gorz and Doogan, namely that they are an individualized reaction to feelings of job insecurity. As Gorz explains, if we feel as though we are in direct competition with colleagues and others for scarce posts of employment then it is little wonder that we will do all we can to impress upon employers our instrumental worth to them – prompting long working hours and the phenomenon of 'presenteeism' (Johns, 2010).

A participant working in the independent media sector reported that he regularly works late into the night and suggested that unrealistic timescales promised to clients by media company 'pitchers' contributed significantly to time pressure:

> There's quite a bit of stress particularly on the short-term jobs, small jobs; quick turnaround basically . . . [if] it's badly priced or something so that the actual pitch has been done for a certain price and a certain time and actually they were over-promising something. (TV and Film Graphic Artist)

Whilst most interviewees that talked in any detail about this issue viewed it as a negative or regrettable phenomenon not everybody did. A university researcher from London suggested that there is trade off between occasionally working longer than contracted hours to militate against feelings of anxiety and that this is a matter of choice:

> I think for me it's much more self-directed, so I will work longer than my contracted hours, but in the majority of cases that's my choice because I am setting myself goals that I need to work an extra hour to achieve, so although it's more pressure I think it makes it easier to accept. If you choose to work longer hours then you can't therefore be unhappy about it, it's your decision isn't it? (University Researcher)

Whilst this was not a widespread view when people were referring to stress in particular, but as will be illustrated in chapter 6, interviewees were more comfortable accepting responsibility for a 'work/life' balance.

The interesting thing however is that according to our data this is most acutely felt by those that are charged with a duty of managing others or are working relatively autonomously – for example freelance workers.

It was generally the case that the more autonomy a person felt they had in their role the more pressure they felt to work longer hours. Whilst this was not associated by any of our participants as a trade off between autonomy and long working hours it is worth noting that they appeared to go hand-in-hand.

Technology

A key component in the changing conditions of work for many people that we spoke to was the role of information technologies. Traditional labour is characterized largely by blue and white collar labour being relatively static and confined to prescribed hours of work (Grint, 2005). For many of the people that we interviewed this was not their experience. The part that technology plays however, was not only seen as significant by those who had been in the labour market for a period of time – and had experienced change – but also those relatively new to work. The key impact of information technologies was the extension of the working day. The idea of flexible working is often touted as a positive attribute of utilizing new technologies but many of the people that we spoke to thought that this 'flexibility' opened up the possibilities for increased demands from employers and even prohibition. A health service employee suggested that the use of mobile phones and e-mail simply increased expectations of availability:

> I think as IT progresses and the fact that no one actually switches off their mobile phone anymore like they did two or three years ago . . . I mean, I wouldn't have dreamt of turning on my mobile phone at weekends or in the evening a few years ago . . . I think with Blackberry – I call it Crackberry, it never gets turned off! But I also think that once you hit a particular level in an organization there is an expectation that you will be available much more than just 9 to 5. (Health Service Manager)

A worker in education accentuated the deadening effect of an over reliance on machines to deliver what is essentially a human activity – productive labour:

> I don't use a blackberry actually because I think it makes you even more of a slave. I think e-mail, we were only having a discussion recently actually about this at senior leadership team, that you can end up, I mean on the downside that you can actually end up just being responsive all the time rather than sitting or rather being creative yourself and actually setting the agenda and you sort of having the vision, you end up just sort of responding all the time and reacting to e-mails and . . . you know obviously we need to set the agenda and you answer e-mails at the end of the week or . . . you know rather than feeling that you have to be online 24/7. (Assistant Head Teacher)

It is interesting that this interviewee associated information technology as stifling elements of creativity within their work. For us this echoes the view that Gorz offers of capitalist labour markets that celebrate the idea of creativity and autonomy without being able to deliver them – or what Gorz calls 'autonomy within heteronomy' (1997: p. 39). There were many more comments on the expectation of availability online or by telephone and most saw this as a bad thing. There were a couple of instances where interviewees reflected on the usefulness to them of using technologies in ways that they hadn't previously considered. There was an example of an administrator that decided that they could compartmentalize all of the tasks of their job that involved being online into one day and then need not waste time travelling. There was also this example from a researcher:

> In terms of when I was researching . . . [I] started using my blog in a very particular way and you know some people don't, it's a chore for them and they don't enjoy it but I quite enjoy writing. I quite enjoy using that as a focus point for me to move out from and you know then drop links into my blog or whatever . . . a big part of my job is trying to use new technologies in that kind of way, you know to interact with people at a distance. (Academic Researcher)

It is interesting to note that one of the few people that felt they were reaping rewards from using new technologies was employed to explore the potential of new technologies, but also that some of his colleagues saw it as a 'chore' – despite being in an environment that valued new technologies as potentially beneficial they still found aspects of using them of no value.

Anxiety/Stress

For Baldamus the concept of fatigue was particularly pertinent as in 1961 this was perceived as an overriding cause of dissatisfaction with work. It is interesting to note that its modern corollary, stress, shares many features – particularly in its ubiquitous use. Baldamus uses an explanation of fatigue as subjectively constituted and 'the feeling of the individual being unpleasantly tired unable to enjoy his evening of leisure, feeling discontented with a life which requires him to work until he develops these unpleasant feelings' (Baldamus, 1961: p. 66). Like Baldamus we are interested in the discursive construction of difficulties experienced by people at work and the reasons they give for particular feelings towards these experiences – as Baldamus notes the pervasive nature of 'fatigue' as a catch all, we might do the same with notions of 'stress'.

However, this does not mean that suffering from 'stress' was not seen as generally legitimate or real. This was well iterated by a shop worker in our interview data who said that a consequence of a business not doing well was that people suffer:

> Well I guess in the worst case scenario people could be off sick. They could be off sick with genuine things, like stress, or in the worst case depression. (Shop Worker)

Some of our interviewees identified it as the main concern in relation to well-being at work, but importantly that it was relational. A clerical assistant suggested that it was the key contributor to unhappiness at work saying possible causes in her field as 'being overworked and underpaid . . . mainly being pushed beyond limits' and later in her interview: 'I'd say stress is the most important thing' (Clerical Assistant). As is suggested in these interviews experiences of stress related to many different aspects of people's lives, some of which have been mentioned earlier – long hours of work and negative relationships at work, but these relationships take many forms. A worker in a call centre identified the fleeting relationships she has with the general public as a key factor in her experience of stress, saying that she had to 'deal with people who are unhappy on the phone' and what she euphemistically referred to as 'different situations', implying that these situations were often not enjoyable or fulfilling (Call Centre Operative).

The ways in which interviewees organized issues of stress and the concomitant personal relationships were along hierarchical lines on the one hand (managers, the public, etc) and peer lines on the other (co-workers, other employees). An interesting insight into relationship management and management of one's own stress came in an interview with a factory machinist. Whilst he acknowledged the role of other's performance at work as being a contributory factor in his own stress, he also accentuated the role of respect and status. When asked what sort of things prevent people being happy at work he replied 'I'd say people not working as a team. They'd try to do things on their own, trying to get credit for things on their own, not passing the credit on, things like that', (Factory Machinist). He then immediately moves the discussion on to stress summarizing his feelings about what makes a person 'stressed' at the end of this passage of the interview

'... what you have on board, what you have to do yourself, what your job title is, things like that...' (Factory Machinist). This was reiterated by a retail worker who suggested that not being recognized for work that she considered commensurate with a higher position in the shop was a cause of stress (Retail Assistant). This is a theme that is picked up later in the book with reference to the relationship between line managers and senior managers, but it is worth noting at this stage that there has been work, particularly in higher education and nursing that has identified lack of recognition and reward as a major contributory factor in individual experiences of work related stress (Gillespie *et al.*, 2001: p. 64–65; Sengin, 2003).

Another interviewee acknowledged that performance-related inducements for productivity are a cause of anxiety and stress in a job market where insecurity is a key characteristic of many people's perceptions of their working lives (Worker in Construction) – clearly indicative of the point made by Doogan about manufactured insecurity (Doogan, 2009: p. 194).

One way of interpreting these accounts is to view them in isolation, or as individual experiences that are more or less mediated through relationships that are not necessarily universal. However, we would argue that the conditions for these experiences being so prevalent are culturally mediated and, as is implied by Baldamus, from these individual accounts comes a view of culture operating at both a micro level (what happens to an individual at work) and at a macro level (this seems to be happening to everyone and something is maintaining it). One interviewee, a police officer, specifically refers to 'a culture' implying something that is happening at his work. He said 'a lot of the stress is not post traumatic stress, a lot of it is working long hours, a culture of having to be seen' (Police Officer). This statement, whilst referring to one place of work resonates to many.

Alongside abstract discussions of how and where stress can reside, or questions of well-being, there was acknowledgement that pressure at work can and does directly impact on health. A Senior University Administrator said:

> I was very ill a year ago and that was trying to do two jobs, I was doing [role title] job and my old [role title] job and you don't do that for too long without it impacting on your health, and physically it impacted on me because mentally, mostly, I can actually kind of cope with a fair amount and I know that and I know the boundaries are of it, but eventually, it impacted on my health, so I kind of said 'right I've got to do something about it.' (Senior University Administrator)

A teacher spoke about a former colleague:

> [My] previous boss had a breakdown and had to be literally taken out in an ambulance and then they found bottles of alcohol in his filing cabinet and he was a Deputy Head. (Teacher)

A freelance television graphics designer talked about a colleague that started weeping uncontrollably after a particularly stressful period of work and spoke of another colleague:

> Like a guy I was working with, we were working through the night and stuff and after this little stint of madness we had to do, he got shingles and couldn't go to work for two weeks, and he wouldn't have got that unless he'd been working like a nutter. (Graphic Designer)

As is widely documented our relationship to stress is more complicated, then you have it and then you suffer (Aldwin, 2007; Moos and Schaeffer, 1986). Despite the widespread belief that stress was a key contributor to mental ill health at work amongst our interviewees, there was acknowledgement, that a certain amount of stress is a natural reaction to being at work, as one university manager explained:

> 'Well, I would fully support,' is a normal reaction, actually a very healthy reaction, it's kind of pathological I think when people demonstrate that they are not having the normal responses to help them overcome their stress, or feel that they can't cope in some way. So one example would be a lecturer who burst into tears at every occasion and demonstrates that her responses are not within the normal reactions. (University Manager)

This pathologized narrative was picked up by a university contract researcher when he talked about his initial response to managing the 'natural' stress documented above. He also suggested that people develop strategies for coping with stress but that these are individualized to such an extent that people have trouble identifying whether they are healthy or not:

> I mean, I have in the past managed my stress maladaptively I think, well I know; but you know as one gets older as well I think you perhaps find different ways of, or you don't, of managing stress. I do a lot more exercise now, which I find hugely beneficial. You know, and that's my kind of, that's my

sort of stress relief mechanism, and I'm thinking about yoga and things, and just trying to do things that are, you know, helping to relax I suppose. (University Contract Researcher)

Whilst some managers were sceptical of the prevalence of 'stress' as a feature of modern absenteeism, they still conceded that there was an increase in pressure on workers over time:

Bad back is sort of number two on the list, but number one is now, kind of, stress and depression. Work related stress seems to have come in there as well really, which personally I sort of suspect as being a bit overrated but I am sure that there must be an element of truth in it somewhere. I mean people do feel more stressed in their workplace than they did kind of 10 or 15 years ago. (Civil Service Manager)

Another attributed the highlighting of policies to counter stress at work as actually contributing to the problem. When a particular policy was introduced into her place of work she describes her reaction:

Oh right here we go! We're giving everybody licence to just go 'I feel stressed, I'm going off sick!' You know . . . In certain parts of the Trust there is a culture amongst some staff that once they've used up their annual leave they can then take a couple of weeks off sick from stress. (Health Service Manager)

There has been a huge amount written about stress and work and it is not our contention that much of the literature is incorrect. From our perspective it is clear that stress is experienced – and attributes of stress often have negative connotations for people at work. The ways in which people frame experiences that psychologists might refer to by positive benefits of stress (Aldwin, 2007; Moos and Schaeffer, 1986) are explained in terms of similar sensations – 'adrenaline rush' or excitement, rather than stress. That said it is also clear that 'stress' is understood in different ways by different people. Some saw stress as something akin to an illness while others thought it was something more bogus – a pathology to be exploited by the work-shy. What we also felt became apparent was that stress has a discursive, almost performative element. Once again we should say that this is not to undermine people's experience of the phenomena but as is illustrated in the quote comparing stress as the modern bad back it has come to be understood as a distinct experience through knowledge of it. As way of illustration inputting the search terms 'work employment stress' into the search engine google scholar[3] returns 3270 articles between 1950 and 1959, 14 600 articles between 1970 and 1979, 53 700 articles between 1990 and 1999 and 172 000 articles between 2000 and 2009. Whilst this is by no means scientific it does indicate an increased level of interest in the subject – as well as perhaps the increase in academic published material more generally. However we wish to frame stress, people are keen to point out that it is caused by external factors. Whilst some people might be described as 'highly strung' it is only through our reaction to circumstances that stress can be identified. For a study of work and employment it was clear, as is illustrated throughout the book, that there were structural factors that could account for many of the negative feelings people had at work.

Relationships/Perception of Others

A key factor in people's reporting of their experiences of work is relationships with others. These were talked about hypothetically as good or bad, and presented by participants as integral to their own orientations to their actual jobs.

> I'd say the top thing was work colleagues. This can have a big impact on how someone feels at work. Obviously in work relationships you deal with those people most of your working days so that's obviously a big thing. But also I think obviously how you are treated, say for instance by customers has a big impact. (Shop Worker)

When asked what made them happy at work positive friendly relationships were identified by almost all of our interviewees irrespective of sector or hierarchical position. For example a wood machinist when asked what made him happy at work replied the friends that he had made in his job (Wood Machinist), a shop worker suggested that other people getting on was key (Shop Worker). A university researcher said:

> I think working relationships are so important, I really do. I think they're probably the most important thing because even if everything else is getting you down at work, if you have a bit of fun, chat, and can laugh it off with

---

[3] This trawl was performed in 'advanced scholar search' selecting articles only from social sciences, arts and humanities.

colleagues, that makes it a lot better. So I think poor working relationships are definitely a big one. I know I keep saying that but I just think that it's important. (Academic Researcher)

A sales manager when asked what made him happy at work said 'good atmosphere, cheery atmosphere when you come in, in the mornings. Good bit of a laugh, bit of a craic' (Sales Manager). The centrality of good relationships with people at work was recognized by all of our interviewees – as was the centrality of bad working relationships to damaging a sense of well-being. In the interviews the perceptions our colleagues have of us and each other appeared to be important for understanding legitimacy and culture. This was best exampled when people spoke about colleagues that had been unwell and the judgements they faced if it were deemed that their illness was unreasonable to the culture of work established in any particular environment. Whilst supportive relationships were good and contributed to a sense of worth and well-being, there were corrosive elements to the ways in which people experienced or exacted judgements on others. Whilst many assumed that their co-workers would be supportive of somebody struggling with mental health issues others did not. One civil servant said 'I think there is a lot less understanding. I think sometimes there is a lot of resentment' (Civil Servant). Another used an example that we heard many times in different forms:

> I had a young chap who went off on what we term as long term sickness, which is more than 28 days, I think he had about 28 days with stress and depression. And basically we sort of saw, he lived locally, he was kind of seen in the high street, but you know he hadn't broken his leg, you know, I'm sure he could go out to Woolworths if he wanted to, you know. But he couldn't sort of manage the sort of machinations of what we were doing . . . the medical opinion was that he couldn't come to work. But he was kind of seen and spotted and colleagues didn't like that very much and sort of said, you know 'well if he's well enough you know, I saw him in the pub the other night and he's well enough to be there.' (Civil Servant)

A manager in the health service said:

> Mostly the non-clinical staff have a 'not in my back yard' mentality, which is actually they don't want someone working. (Health Service Manager)

Whilst there is another chapter dealing specifically with experiences of managers an obvious relationship that can have a dramatic effect on feelings of well-being at work is with those that manage. How we are managed is a central feature of our feelings towards our jobs and for most of our interviewees were not always positively experienced:

> Things that make me unhappy? I'd say maybe managers that I don't generally get on with, they may annoy me and try and stress me out maybe. (Retail Outlet Supervisor)

Another interviewee summed up what many others said:

> Mainly at work I'd say if I'm not supported by managers and things like that. If there's no support. (Customer Service Advisor)

It appeared as though there were certain expectations that managers and staff being managed had of each other's roles that made a conflict inevitable – and again these could be read as culturally bound. The ways in which career progression works in managerial positions was condemned by one interviewee who was herself a manager but felt as though her progression would be hampered by her unwillingness to behave like some of her peers:

> That's when careerist issues become a problem, I don't get a name by changing a few things and making the world a better place to work in necessarily, I get a name if I completely transform the Faculty into something it wasn't before. (University Manager)

The issue of the individualism indicative of careerism is one that Gorz is explicitly concerned with, where the idea that it is not in solidarity that security will be found but in an individualism that is expressed through pursuing goals and aims that are predefined by the employer. This exacerbates a view of incommensurate differences between people working in the same place particularly between ranks or grades in a workplace hierarchy. A consequence of this expectation of managerialist individualism is that, even when people's behaviour is not deliberately motivated by self-interest it is perceived as such by others. A worker in the civil service gave an illustration of this when talking about issues of confidentiality:

> It plays out by people saying 'you're not transparent, why don't you tell us, because then we'd understand?' And you just have to say 'I cannot tell you, you just have to trust me there are very good reasons . . .' Being trustworthy,

that you have to say to people 'there are good reasons but I can't share them' that's all you can do really, and hope for the level of trust from colleagues that your own reputation is sufficient and superior so they all know to shut up really. (Civil Servant)

The bottom line for this worker is that their place in the hierarchy and the perception of them as (a) someone that can be trusted and (b) someone who's reputation is 'superior' should be enough to garner an environment where there is a lack of trust because of secrecy. The point here is that the cultural interpretation of the role of manager is one who is not to be trusted, and the resolution for this particular individual is that their personal behaviour and reputation can overcome this cultural preconception. As will be illustrated in the next section, the conflict between the process of subjection and prohibitive cultures of work are decisive factors in the pervasive sense of lack of fulfilment that so many people appear to experience whilst at work.

It became clear throughout the interviews that in larger organizations a deferment of decision-making or intervention to personnel or occupational health departments was widespread, and that this provided some protection or re-assurance to managers in particular when dealing with employees. One health service worker explained a process where they were obliged to introduce occupational health if they felt a person was struggling:

> Basically, it comes down to if you've done everything possible that you can, saying 'I think you're unwell, I would like to be able to support you with this. Have you been to your GP? Have you got friends? Have you got a support network? Can we refer you to occupational health? Actually as a manager, I have to refer you to occupational health.' And then you get 'no,' they're fine, because the person actually presents ok, and is able to manage it. You're absolutely stuffed, you're stuffed, because then, if you have worries about their practice and their fitness to practise you then have to go through occupational health HR disciplinary hearing. (Health Service Manager)

Whilst the principle appears on the surface to be reasonable it concealed a great deal. First is that there is the recourse to insisting that an employee receive support is punitive. This appears to undermine the principle of support or care. Another issue for some of our interviewees was the translation of advice from personnel or occupational health to the work situation. As a University Manager explained:

> Personnel are there to advise you, but at the end of the day they're often not in the room when you're faced with the person in whatever condition they're in and you have to respond humanely in all of those situations and as a manager, it's a one way street and sometimes that's very testing on human beings, because we're all human beings at the end of the day. (University Manager)

So there is a depersonalization from the mechanism of support – the manager has to refer a problem to the support division and then is tasked with the duty of carrying out the support recommended.

One element that emerged from interviews with people in large organizations was the franchising out of institutional mechanisms of support. Many places had access to occupational health support but this was being provided by an external agency that was being bought in by the organization. What is particularly interesting about this is the ongoing logic of the depersonalization of support. Occupational health as an occasional intervention already provides a distance from a person that might be struggling or need assistance at work from a highly personal intervention from their own manager for example. The manager can introduce a distant intervention from a person previously unknown to the employee. In this sense the occupational health worker provides an arbitration of the emotional involvement between the employee and their manager – clearly making it easier for the manager to represent an institutional response to the problems of the employee – as is illustrated in the example above where the manager was duty bound to bring in occupational health if an employee was perceived to be suffering from stress related problems. By franchising occupational health out of the organization into the hands of an entirely separate entity the process of depersonalization continues. The institutional response to the problems of an employee no longer runs the risk of an internal conflict – for example an occupational health division failing to agree with another internal division that a particular course of action is appropriate in dealing with employees.

Goal Orientation/Achievement

It has long been recognized that having a clear, achievable set of objectives at work is important for maintaining a sense of worth and well-being at work (see for example ter Doest et al., 2006; Macdonald et al., 2006:

p. 118–24). It is certainly the case in our study that employees felt that they needed a sense of purpose and goals that were attainable and this was important to them. These goals tended to be set by the organization and, through a managerial structure, were filtered down. There were very occasional instances where interviewees suggested they were responsible for setting their own targets – and those that did were freelance workers who later suggested that they were on very tight targets but could choose their jobs and people that had a degree of flexibility in how they achieved particular goals or targets for example researchers and self-employed people. On the whole individual's targets or objectives appear to be set alongside larger corporate targets or objectives – and this should be no surprise. It also chimes nicely with the idea that what is good for the company or organization is good for the individual. For Gorz this sense of worth through contemporary work leads to subjection. If the worker comes to define their worth through validation of achievements at work that are defined solely through corporate objectives their sense of worth as a worker is in some senses owned by those setting the objectives. For us this is a neoliberal mythology that suggests that it is possible to satisfy both individual and corporate aspirations harmoniously – and that the two are synonymous.

Throughout the interviews we noticed a fluctuation between the personal and the corporate, and these apparently shared principles were important to people. The idea that people were doing either a worthwhile job or doing a job well was represented as being an important part of feeling good at work. In the private sector, the owner of a construction business said that the setting of objectives was good for his workers:

> We've tried not to be too intense at [name of firm] and coming back to that reason, that if at the end of the day, if you don't wake up feeling that you want to go to do your job, then it's not much in the way of satisfaction that can be gained from that. You also have to try and set a ladder so that people can see where they are going, they have clear objectives and goals set and they can see a way forward and improvement in their life over time. And that's what we try to do so that trying to keep away the stresses and strains. (Office Manager at Building Merchants)

One university manager suggested that not being able to be explicit about the corporate objectives and whether people were satisfying them was a problem:

> I think actually people want to know that they're doing a good job, or that they need to work a bit harder in their particular area. We aren't allowed within the HEI (Higher Education Institutions) though to go into any kind of performance management, so any notion that out of the admin view we would be able to set standards, don't go there. (University Manager)

The primacy of the value of work to individuals is demonstrated by a worker in the voluntary sector:

> Human contact, self esteem, opportunities to build competence, it's a focus, takes you away from other problems you've got, you get validation as a human being, hopefully if it's a nice work environment you just get the basic sense of being connected with something really useful. (Charity Worker)

So the acknowledgement that work can give us a sense of worth and well-being is widely espoused – and is of course at the centre of the dichotomy addressed in part by this book: Why do people think work is good for themselves and others when they often express how unhappy it makes them? It is perhaps the discourse of neoliberal working that the unholy alliance of individual and corporate objectives being one in the same that creates this disjuncture. They are not the same – the interests of the corporate organization are not implicitly the same as the interests of the individual – and whilst they might often appear to coincide, when they diverge the difference between them becomes clear, a point demonstrated in the swathe of job losses in the UK throughout 2008–2009 (Gregg and Wadsworth, 2010). In Gorz we find the danger of pinning our hopes on the social bonds artificially created within organizations where the demands for flexibility and autonomy are always predicated on predefined corporate objectives and where in the end 'the subject's lifeworld is circumscribed by the company's system of ends and values'(Gorz, 1999: p. 38). This might sound over the top and a criticism of this perspective could be that what we are talking about is simply the difference between good management, or good corporate practice, and bad. However, our contention is that the logic of late industrial capital operates in such a way as to force us to seek happiness where we can in the overarching systems – or machines to paraphrase Illich – in which we operate. It is only human then to find positives in something inherently negative (Baldamus, 1961: p. 7–11).

Alongside positive attributes of working towards goals or objectives, negative aspects of corporate working were expressed and these often exposed the contradiction inherent in assuming individual needs and corporate objectives are intrinsically the same thing. The charity worker quoted above described a working situation that involves:

> ... unreasonable pressures, a not person-centred environment, an environment that's dishonest or ignores human needs, doesn't recognize people's strengths or contributions, doesn't acknowledge people, yes, and I suppose in other sectors huge demands are placed on people and they're meaningless a lot of the time and I think that's soul destroying. (Charity Worker)

A university manager complained that the lack of standards meant that staff were unable to appraise their own performance – but this means that this appraisal can be performed by a manager who will then be able to manage the levels of emotional or social attachment that a member of staff might feel, simply by telling them they are doing a good job or a bad job:

> One goes back to what we were talking about, that none of the administration staff, we ask them 'how do you know you are doing a good job?' because there are no standards set for them. And actually that's quite stressful because you don't know if you're doing it well, you don't know if you're doing it badly. (University Manager)

A worker in the health service, a massive organization, understood that the corporate goals are turned into targets that have to be met, and that the human or altruistic aspects of the job inhabit individuals not the corporate:

> It is the government targets. It's targets, it's weightings, it's ... you know, Health Care Commission. It's everything. It's this constant thing you know, traffic light systems on everything ... it is exhausting actually, and so you have to hold onto, or those of us who, you know, actually still want to try and make a difference in terms of what we are doing for the organization, you know, you have to sort of hold onto that sort of quality issue and keep shouting about it. (Health Service Manager)

The question of motivation and morals also arose in relation to individual and corporate motivations. When talking about senior managers in a particular environment one interviewee suggested that the goal orientation of the organization does not match the moral or ethical values of people that entered it, but after time some people simply adapt to a corporate managerialism at the expense of their ethical orientation:

> I don't think necessarily it's how they came into it, or their core values, but I think core values disappear, because of the fire fighting, the finance, you know, what they have to achieve. (Health Service Manager)

This perception of values or an ethic being subverted by managerialist and economic concerns were fairly widespread. A worker in education made a similar point, but rather than suggesting people changed over time she implied that there are two types of people from the outset:

> In creative disciplines, managerially, there are two types of people. There are people that are grounded, if you like, in practice and there are people who weren't that good at practice and really want to be a manager . . . I feel there's an awful, there's been in academic life, quite a shift in managerial cultures, partly to do with things like universities engaging with business. (University Manager)

The idea of personal and corporate goal orientation and achievement is one that could do with more dedicated critical engagement, however, there was widespread acknowledgement that a sense of purpose was important and without one, work can become onerous, that when corporate objectives match personal objectives people seem to feel good about work but that these crossovers are not commonly experienced. For us it should be no surprise that these crossovers are relatively rare. If we return to Baldamus' view that work is naturally disharmonious then it should be anticipated that the natural state of working environments is that they are riven with discontinuity, compromise and inequity. In order to enable people to feel better about being at work we should attend to those instances where people are reporting happiness – namely where corporate objectives match personal objectives. For us this doesn't involve a recalibration of personal aspiration but an overhaul of employment culture.

Concluding Comments – Cultures of Work

Throughout the interviews it was evident that most people perceived that there had been an intensification of their work and work in general. This was most clearly demonstrated by the extended hours that people reported working, and increased demands made on them by others. This was explained in part by the increasing reliance on information technologies as a component in communicating particular aspects of people's jobs. The elements that do not need face-to-face contact or a material engagement with a workplace can be conducted remotely and, crucially, at any time of the day or night. This increased accessibility means that some employers appeared to be exploiting this to optimize levels of productivity from people – outside of agreed contracted hours. Another key element in this intensification process we would argue is cultural. The expectation that people will work beyond an agreed remit becomes a self-fulfilling prophesy. If, in order to prove competency, an employee has to demonstrate commitment outside of agreed contractual boundaries then this is what they tend to do – particularly in a competitive labour market environment.

Alongside the intensification there appears to us to have been a process of target or objective driven systematization. There was a feeling in the interviews that the space to be creative or aspirational fell between very tight pre-prescribed parameters. In this sense individualism and autonomy were valued in relation to achieving corporate objectives, and only when they tallied with either career aspiration or the bypassing of traditional industrial social bonds – social class for example (not a single interviewee spoke about the importance of trade unions or worker representation). This systematization of work extends into a systematization of individual needs – particularly when problems arise. This was explained by a public sector worker in this way:

> ... we definitely sort of say even within the service 'oh no, you don't need to know anything about empathy, what you need to do is follow the process.' And what we're looking at is a standard operation model and anyone can do that and they don't need to have any special insight or understanding. (Civil Servant)

Despite this systematization the importance of good human relationships was seen by many as key to feeling good about work, however, particular styles of management, for example as described above, seemed to jar with an affective relationship as important. Throughout our interviews the disharmony of work as described by Baldamus was evident, people tended to speak about good practice or good experiences as out of the ordinary or something to be noticed.

The value of the individual relationship, cited by many interviewees as important for feeling good at work, appears to be undermined by the institutional response demanded by the organization. The requirement of a manager – who has a personal relationship with the worker that is struggling – to refer them to occupational health division depersonalizes the process of support or resolution. It is perhaps then to be expected that there is a disenfranchisement of the worker to the process of support – they are treated as a problem to be resolved rather than a person to be supported. It is also a disenfranchisement of the manager as the person responsible for the well-being of the worker – the manager is concerned with corporate objectives not their workers. This is particularly true in those organizations which have franchised out their occupational health divisions. This process reflects the dichotomy highlighted by Illich and Gorz where the increasing non-convivial tendency of employers to treat workers as necessary for the maintenance of a system alongside the debilitating effects of Gorz's subjection – where a worker's social bonds are supported largely within their understanding of their place at work – will only damage the sense of worth, or mental well-being of the worker. It is the modern capitalist contradiction where the illusion of autonomy, freedom and satisfaction offered by post-Taylorism is undermined by the unchanging logic of industrial capital. In their own small way those organizations farming out support to external providers are contributing to the depersonalization of working relations, the very thing people appear to want or need.

As we have suggested there is continuity between how we have worked through the twentieth century and how we work today. We think that the cult of the new sometimes obscures things that we already have answers for. Our use of Baldamus, Illich and Gorz to help us understand contemporary work in the UK and its relationship to mental health is our attempt to point this out. Throughout our data there are allusions from interviewees that they are also aware that whilst some things have changed others have not – and that this is not necessarily in their best interests. An interesting example came from a relatively senior administrator in higher education:

> I think there's more pressure because there's more kinds of monitoring, so there are more kinds of catch points . . . Funnily enough the academic contract, if you just take the contract straight, hasn't changed much at all. (Senior University Administer)

This observation adds a layer of complexity to the increasingly acknowledged view that it is not work that has changed but contracts of employment (Doogan, 2009). However, this observation tends to pertain to tenure rather than what jobs actually involve. Combining these two observations presents a fairly gloomy picture of contemporary employment practice – namely short term contracts are becoming increasingly common and, whilst these contracts may not appear to be different in terms of their definitions of roles, they mask an increasing intensification of work that people feel is detrimental to their well-being. A change in culture does not necessarily require large scale structural change. A senior police officer explained that the fundamental principles and expectations people had of his service had not changed but the culture within policing had:

> You've got a performance culture. A lot of the biggest stresses is that sort of performance culture . . . [a] culture of finger pointing and know your business, which is good – bit of a professional challenge is appropriate – but this league table culture, the winners and losers, the boss phoning you up at two 7 o'clocks in the day, 'I expect you to be there for both of them'! (Police Officer)

The cultural expectations of people whilst they are working are potentially every bit as debilitating as the structural impediments to well-being. From working outside of contracted hours – because that is what happens in a particular workplace – to the distancing of human relationships at work through the franchising out of support in the shape of occupational health or human resources departments. From the disenfranchisement of managers to the judgements made by peers expected to pick up work left by those off sick, the cultures of work that in the twenty-first century are being constructed through an increased reliance on technology, 'efficiency' and working beyond contractual agreements create situations where respite or explanation is found in the identification of and discourse of 'stress'.

Whilst much is made of the ideas of flexibility and autonomy we found little evidence of this either in practice or being celebrated as elements of people's work that made them happy. It is perhaps an expression of autonomous working that people appeared to prefer to imagine that they were not being monitored. At the same time however, they were not suggesting that they were encouraged to think of themselves as autonomous. As for flexibility, it seems to us that this extended in one direction – the employee needs to be flexible to accommodate the 'needs' of the employer. These processes and expectations of work all contribute to what we would call a culture of work. In much the same way as Baldamus we would like to see our approach as being able to accommodate the micro level of individuals in workplaces – and acknowledge that there are unique features in every workplace – that could be argued to contribute to micro cultures, but that the general similarities that we see replicated across sectors and hierarchies contribute to a sense of particular features of working in Britain as universally applicable. The dichotomy between a neoliberal labour market and our experiences of being employed were summed up by a police officer when he explained how he felt his employers viewed him – on the one hand property and on the other autonomous:

> get on with it', it's almost like 'I own you,' like someone would have a go at a professional footballer and say, 'well you're a superstar, you earn this salary, get on with it. (Police Officer)

In terms of our expectations of the interviews that we conducted many were confounded. Two of the most obvious omissions were any real discussion of job security or money worries. It seemed as though these concerns at the beginning of a recession were either too obvious or too frightening to iterate. It is interesting that people, when asked what made them happy at work all highlighted human relationships – perhaps in times of economic hardship we are forced to evaluate what is really important to us.

Chapter 4

Techniques of Identity Governance and Resistance: Formulating the Neoliberal Worker

Carl Walker, Ben Fincham, with Josh Cameron

The ten million people suffering from a mental health problem at any one time are the largest silent minority in the country. (Rt Hon Alan Johnson, Secretary of State for Health, 2008)

While work can be beneficial for people experiencing mental health problems, any construction of the workplace as an unproblematic theatre of recovery lacks the necessary sophistication to understand the lived experiences of mental health service users in work. It is undoubtedly true that there can be multiple benefits that accrue from being able to earn a living wage and from avoiding the painful social isolation that so often accompanies mental health experiences and particularly the time spent on sick leave. However if we leave the story here it is far from complete. For Gorz, the experiences of subjection that are so characteristic of modern employment have fashioned workers who have been stripped of the social identities that protected them against the debilitating effects of capitalist social relations (Gorz, 1999).

In an era when workers are encouraged to gauge their self-worth through the relationship with their employer or firm, the paradoxical relationship between work and mental health status is particularly problematic. There has been ample research that has documented the very common and insidious experiences of stigma and discrimination that are commonplace for many people with mental health problems at work. This makes an uncritical subscription to the 'work as recovery' discourse all the more difficult. There is an undoubted complexity in the way that mental health is experienced at work and this is especially salient in this era of neoliberal capitalist social relations where the modern workplace demands an autonomous subject that copes with any conditions thrown at it (Gill, 2008; Walkerdine, 2002).

This complexity relates to potentially damaging work environments dominated by increased drives for productivity and concomitant rises in work intensity. Environments marked by general increases in job insecurity and the flexibilization of labour; of experiences of resentment, discrimination and abuse. However there are also the wholly beneficial accounts of positive experiences, of feeling useful, of being around friends and colleagues, of continuing to be able to have access to essential commodities. Very often these experiences co-occur both in workplaces and in the narratives of individual people experiencing mental health difficulties and this complexity means that the relationship between work and mental health is both multifaceted and contradictory. The mainstream UK political parties have, thus far, largely unpacked this beguiling convolution by setting up camp in the 'work as beneficial' side of the debate and so much of recent policy and practices have tended to be framed by discourse that represents work as, if not essential, then certainly facilitative of recovery. And while there is a detailed research literature on the abject experiences of degradation and inequity for those mental health service users who continue to attend the workplace, very little of this research has adequately been able to capture the multiplicity of social relations and discursive labour that frame the working lives of people with mental health problems.

It is common for both the stigma research and the 'work benefit' research (for they rarely coexist in the literature) to represent the person with a mental health problem as an object to which others respond through comments, actions and in some cases, inaction. Definitions of mental health and the identities of people with mental health problems, colleagues, managers and supervisors are often posited as fixed and invariable. There has been little attention paid to the social processes, practices and relationships through which identities are negotiated, constructed and fixed, nor the way that they vary depending on both the symbolic and material resources available in given work environments.

There has been little focus on the way that configurations of work and the personhood of certain workers comes to be problematized, nor the social labour that recreates local truths about the ways in which working lives should be conducted (Miller and Rose, 2008). It is only by understanding these processes and their relationships to the prevailing and dominant cultures of work that we can try to understand the lived experiences of being a working person with mental health difficulties or indeed a known mental health history. Workplaces are, first and foremost, sites of economic and material production and, as such, are spaces for processes of domination, sometimes subtle, sometimes less so. Moreover, these processes of domination and control produce particular types of human subjectivity, subjectivities that come to be 'owned' by the people who live within the bounds of these systems (Deetz, 1997). That is, until, as happens with those experiencing mental ill health, actors are unable to operate within the given and accepted subject spaces. In so many organizations the identities of mental health and ill health directly contradict pervasive and dominant forms of rational production and so become sites of discursive reproduction, negotiation and conflict. As Deetz noted of modern corporations:

> ... central though is an understanding of the relations among power, discursive practices and conflict suppression as they relate to the production of individual identity and corporate knowledge. (Deetz, 1992: p. 22)

Knight and Wilmott state that:

> ... sense of subjectivity or self-consciousness is a product of the involvement in relations of power through which conceptions of identity are generated. (Knight and Wilmott, 1989: p. 537)

Moreover,

> ... the meanings of and membership within the categories of discursive practice will be a constant site of struggle over power as identities become posited, resisted and fought over. (Clegg, 1997: p. 29)

Drawing on Foucault, Miller and Rose (2008: p. 16) outline the key role of technologies of government and performance, '... assemblages of persons, techniques, institutions, instruments for the conducting of conduct' that permit certain ways of rendering problems thinkable and knowable in the workplace. Much of the research on people who experience mental health problems at work fails to provide an adequate account of the way that discrimination and inequality involve struggles of power that are, in so many cases, struggles of identity.

It is these very processes and techniques that are key in reconfiguring identities that fail to submit to the logic of naturalized axiomatic notions of what it means to be a good employee. The institutionalized premise of neoliberal capitalism provides powerful discourses that promote acceptable employee identities as self-regulating individuals at the mercy, not of circumstance, but of deliberative choice; as intentional narrators of their own lives (Gill, 2008) that become naturalized and taken for granted. These constraints in 'ways of being' are manifest in identity negotiation and normalizing judgements that act as efficient means of controlling and regulating conduct. It is these very sites of political struggle between different actors striving to realize their ambitions that so much of the work on occupational mental health experiences fails to adequately address. We sympathize with Knights and Wilmott (1989) in noting that, thus far, there has been too little attention given to the way that modes of management control reproduce very particular identities and subjectivities in the workplace.

Techniques of power develop to meet the specific demands of production in modern workplaces (Jackson and Carter, 1997) and it is the manifestations of these techniques of power, and the ways in which they are resisted, subverted and directly contested that forms the base of this chapter. Thornicroft (2006) noted that 47% of mental health service users described experiences of discrimination at work. Thomas and Secker (2005) found that 78% of service users reported having lost one or more jobs as a result of mental ill-health. Irvine (2008) showed that line managers often found it difficult to understand the nature of mental health recovery. This work is essential but it doesn't provide an account of the everyday discursive, rhetorical and relational processes and practices, and of the associated techniques of power demanded by modern neoliberal capitalism, which frame the development of the deviant, illegitimate or stigmatizable identities extant in modern working cultures. For us, Eakin's (2005) contention that people returning to work from mental ill-health are required to 'perform' their credibility and integrity acts as an invitation to open up a new avenue of inquiry that places institutionalized workplace practices, social performance and identity work at the centre of the way we understand the lived experiences of mental ill-health at work.

From the Global to the Local – A Study of Work and Mental Health in South East England

Our own data, with a number of employees in the South East of England, support the contention that people with mental health difficulties have a number of problematic experiences in work. For this chapter we undertook detailed semi-structured interviews with 20 current or former mental health service users in the South East of England area. Our participants varied in their employment status at time of interview. A few participants were employed but the majority were either unemployed or on short or long-term sick leave. Participants were recruited from two sources. Seven participants were recruited from acute mental health services (either inpatient of Crisis resolution or Home Treatment Teams) from two sites of one mental health trust in England. There were four men and three women and their ages ranged between 21 and 45. All were white British. None of these participants considered that they had a disability although the interviews suggest that their symptoms would meet the medical criteria for major depression, bipolar disorder and psychosis.

The remaining thirteen participants were recruited from an employment and mental health project that was run by a mental health charity in the South East of England. People could be referred by their GP (the main source), health workers, employers or could self-refer. The project mainly worked with people by providing support and interventions from a project worker on an individual basis (usually involving their employers) but it also provided a monthly evening support group facilitated by a project worker.

These participants reported receiving a range of mental health diagnoses (including depression, bipolar disorder, and schizo-affective disorder) which most had experienced as recurring or enduring conditions. Most were being supported for their mental health problems by primary care services, though some were currently receiving input from specialist mental health services. There were nine women and four men aged between 29 and 54 (average 42.5). Eleven were single, one married and one had a non-cohabiting partner. All were White British.

It is difficult to know the proportion of people nationwide whose experiences match those of our participants below, especially since it is possible that our project participants' employment experiences may have been more likely to have been problematic. However, the extensive work which outlines the prevalent nature of stigmatizing and discriminating encounters at work in the UK (Eakin, 2005; Seebohm, 2005; Stuart, 2004; Thomas and Secker, 2005; Thornicroft, 2006) suggests that the events that we outline below are far from uncommon.

Adjustments

Although the majority of the experiences that participants relayed were problematic and distressing, there were encounters that were undoubtedly positive for the service users and certainly supported suggestions that the workplace was not only useful as a means of reducing the isolation and financial encroachments of being off work, but could also represent a key element in the users' recovery. Indeed the following quote supports Secker, Grove and Membrey's (2005) contention that work should be seen as a significant stage in the journey toward recovery rather than recovery as a precondition to work:

> So there was that ... people were able to sort of see the change in me and ... they ... they were very supportive, they became very supportive, um ... and there was no judgement, which was nice. Because usually if you're off sick for a month or so, you usually get some kind of comment or ... or other such ... such conversations, you know, which aren't very nice. But this ... this workplace have been fantastic, they've been really good. Um ... I'm currently doing um ... sort of rehabilitation into the workplace where I do two days this week, three days next week and then the week after, a full week, so it's re-integrating me slowly. (Assembly Operator)

> I think the first phased return was managed really, really well, and I was given an excellent Practice Manager who was really open and honest with me and would say to me 'actually Marie, you don't seem to be functioning'... and I could talk openly with him about how I felt and he would be able to say to me 'well Marie, you know, if you need to take some TOIL or come in later, whatever, to prevent you taking any time off sick'.... And he was absolutely marvellous and I had him for about two years and I had no time off sick during that time to do with my mental health and in fact to the point where I was promoted to Senior Social Worker. (Senior Social Worker)

A number of participants reflected that first reactions to their mental health problems were often initially positive and it was not uncommon to experience a sense of support at the beginning of their mental health difficulties, before the scale of the difficulties and the support that would potentially be necessary became apparent

> Initially I felt I was being supported. I mean what subsequently happened, was 'cos, I mean I don't know if you, if you want me to go into that but . . . (Administrator)

> At first everyone was very kind and understanding, very gentle with you but then started to notice I wasn't invited to . . . social things. (Care Worker)

This initial support often took the form of line managers and supervisors taking control of the work recovery process in such a way as to implement an *ad-hoc* adjustment process. Although there is plentiful research on some of the problems that many line managers have with both levels of mental health literacy and capacity to understand the needs of their employees with mental health problems (Irvine, 2008), there is little doubt that, since the inception of the Disability Discrimination Act in 1995 and the cascading of health and safety discourses through many industries, the need for adjusted work patterns are often in some way acknowledged. However as the following chapter shows, attending fully to such legislatively enshrined rights is a luxury that few managers could afford. More often than not these *ad-hoc* structural adjustments lacked either the resources and/or the will to maintain them on the part of the line manager and either fell away or never actually happened.

> Yeah, I mean what subsequently happened was that I was sort of continuing to struggle umm, but my, my Manager had said 'what we'll do is we'll have a meeting every, every – it was either every week or every two weeks – to see how you're getting on.' Now that never happened. (Administrator)

The accounts of some service users certainly suggest that in a number of cases there was a proactive recognition of an employee struggling with the demands of their workload and their mental health, and certainly elements of good intent in removing a part of the workload from that employee, but too often the lack of structured framework for this meant that such interventions were insufficient. There was also a perception that, once this *ad-hoc* and usually insufficient intervention was in place, the manager had met their employees' needs. Furthermore, any further or prolonged mental health difficulties would be out of that manager's hands and to a degree beyond their responsibility. When sickness relationships were at this stage, there appeared to be little conflict or negotiation over identities or roles as the relationship was characterized by a seemingly appropriate benevolent endeavour on the part of line managers. However, this approach could prove problematic as staged returns, often conflicted with productivity imperatives and it was not uncommon for this process of staged return or adjustments to be inappropriate or to conclude abruptly and prematurely.

> So I went back to work and we did this staged return and I'd initially sort of said that I feel that I could do X hours for X number of days first, and then build it up but I don't want to push myself past 3 full days until I can see how that's going to be. They said ok, then started to push harder for 'ok, come on, you've got to start increasing your hours now' so I, without really feeling able to, built my hours back up to 4 days. I knew I couldn't go back to 5; it just wasn't going to happen without me becoming seriously unwell. It was a 'this is a full-time job, that's it, end of story' kind of situation. I mean I hadn't even gone back up to the 5 days. It was such a struggle doing the 4 days. I started losing masses of faith in my ability. (NHS Worker)

> Up in London it was, I just had to work and the only arrangements that were made to me, for me, were that I could stay in the office, and have work to do in the office, which wasn't particularly helpful. (Educational Psychologist)

Even this set of limited and potentially damaging circumstances was not available to a number of participants where the notion of adjustment was anathema to the culture of the organization. Mental health was not framed as an appropriate reason to facilitate a reduced workload or time spent in the organization, despite often prolonged sickness absences. In some cases a binary between either being sick or well was constructed and used in such a way as to limit the ways in which the worker could experience their mental illness at work. Such approaches manifestly fail to capture the dynamic variability in subjective wellness of living with a mental illness. This binary is the first instance that we came across where struggles of power were represented as struggles of identity (Knights and Wilmott, 1989), that is, where the interests of the organization were clearly perceived to be best served by failing to allow any identity of sickness that varied between this binary of sick/not sick.

> I wasn't offered it before, I mean I was off . . . two and a half months, but I wasn't offered it before to go back gradually. I just went straight back to my

hours and straight back to my responsibilities just . . . just like that, which probably didn't prove that successful. (Bank Worker)

No, they weren't sort of saying come in a couple of hours a day or anything, they just said you either come back or you're sick, you can't do both. (Postman)

They should have made a reasonable adjustment because they said 'your job is not part-time it's full-time. Therefore, you can't come back to it if you can only do part-time'. So they closed that door, they said no. (NHS Worker)

Umm, so it was very satisfying when I went to the stage one grievance to be able to produce an email that said 'I feel thoroughly depressed and miserable, I need to take some TOIL!' [Laughs]. And what they also had to acknowledge was that no Manager did nothing about that and there was a week when they should have put extra support in place for me, made reasonable adjustments, DDA, they'd known this since 2001. (Senior Social Worker)

The presence of *ad-hoc* accommodations and arrangements on the part of employers could be problematic. A failure on the part of an employee to benefit and recover to their previous status as a healthy productive employee could facilitate a basis to change the identity of the worker, from someone who had mental health problems and who was in the process of returning to wellness, to someone who had been given ample opportunity to recover and remain at work but who refused to or who was beyond the assistance of the company. For some this could signal the beginning of processes of negotiation and conflict regarding the sickness identity of the worker. This often opened up a context to draw upon a discourse of malingering that created a construction of the worker based on their failure to adapt to sympathetic circumstances and hence 'become' unemployable. It also commonly set the scene for a number of practices inexorably driven by the tension between capital and labour and played out in conflicting representations of the worker's sickness identity.

Sick Identities and Patrolling Organizational Subject Spaces

Very often in the case of our participants, work was not only perceived as the source of their mental health difficulties but a contributory hindrance to their recovery as people battled against discrimination and line managers who were unsympathetic or unable to offer sympathy due to the nature of the pressing constraints on their productivity. What we account for as sickness identities resonates with Talcott Parson's (1951) 'sick role', a term used by people regarding the social element of their illness and used as a mechanism for being legitimately excused one's usual duties and, crucially, to be considered not responsible for this. For such an identity to be bestowed, or indeed accepted, by an organization would have considerable financial implications for the organizations. If it were to be accepted that an employee was sick and that they were to be excused culpability for their illness then the organization had little option with regards to the management of what is a difficult situation in a competitive market. Such acceptance for many corporations means that they stand to lose, in the shape of sickness absence, a portion of their productivity and that they have to continue to finance this loss through sick pay. A decision has to be made regarding possible temporary replacements, which represents a further debilitating financial circumstance.

As a way to combat and resist repetitions of this scenario, sickness identities relating to mental health were closely monitored in order to ensure that such identities met the needs of the organization where possible. As Knights and Willmott (1989) note, life at work is dominated by institutional and interpersonal confirmations of social identity, by techniques of identity government that render workers knowable in only certain ways (Miller and Rose, 2008). As a result of the increasing pressures to maintain productive output from their departments we found evidence of managers, colleagues and interviewees negotiating the way that sickness identities could be expressed. Indeed, there was a distinct policing and patrolling of discourses of acceptability that constructed the participant's options regarding sick leave, recovery and ability to do the job. For instance, pressure could emanate from pre-emptive dialogue that implicitly but not explicitly limited the positioning of the sick role. One worker recalled a conversation following a fractious meeting with her manager (Joan) during a time of deteriorating mental health.

> I said 'Oh Joan, I'm afraid that I may be coming depressed again' and she said 'oh Julie (a colleague) already told me' and just carried on with what she was saying'. (Administrator)

Examples like this highlight the fact that managerial responses can open up or indeed close down spaces where sickness identities can be negotiated.

In this case the continuation of the conversation left no space for the depression to be discussed and certainly not as an issue relevant to work. This example of what Goffman (1959) called 'terminating replies' has been reflected in the work of Harkness *et al.* (2005) and is an expression of Deetz's (1997: p. 153) 'closure of responsive options', where disciplining social arrangements produce – a subject aware of the way that the foreclosure of discussions signal their lack of necessity and importance. This has the effect of minimizing and marginalizing the felt distress of the participant and represents a clear closing down of a possible subject space – that of a valid and distressed sufferer of mental ill health. In an almost identical scenario, this event is also reflected in the experience of the following worker:

> During that time, during that supervision session I said, 'Oh actually Cath (supervisor), I'm afraid that I may be becoming depressed again' and she said 'Oh Ruth already told me' and just carried on with what she was saying. (Senior Social Worker)

In the example below there was little discussion of the nature of the participant's problems or indeed the potential for a sickness identity that may occur over a longer term. The suggestion of the mental health problem and medication as being 'short-term' was stated in such a way that anything other than this would be problematic for the organization, participant or both.

> And I said 'look if you can get my bag to me I've got some tablets in there that I can take' so she went out of the room, brought my bag back, gave me the tablets and I took one and she said 'what's that?' and I said 'oh it's Diazepam' she said 'what are you taking those for?' and I said 'it's to help me with my anxiety Julie'. 'In the short-term? I hope it's a short-term thing'? (Senior Social Worker)

> ... when I did approach my line manager and I said that ... Paul makes me more stressed and also that the outcomes, I have to be sure that the outcome doesn't go into a downward spiral and she was really kind of funny about that in her response to me. She was a bit sort of like ... well. ... And it made me frightened to develop my, to develop the point really because I didn't like her response. She just seemed a bit kind of ... like 'well too bad' almost. (Librarian)

This was another example of a manager creating a certain conversational space that limited the acceptable responses from the employee, for them only to be able to respond in certain ways. Here it was clear that the manager's response had denied the employee access to a medical discourse in order to frame her experience. The perception of the employee was that her experience should be constructed as a minor occurrence, a small and unimportant event not worthy of further discussion rather than a conversation about mental ill health that could potentially benefit from a sympathetic but costly set of accommodations. Trying to explain the experience in the first instance received a relatively hostile response which set the boundaries for future dialogue, and hence their possible identity as someone who is sick. Her fear at further developing her point meant that advertently or inadvertently her manager patrolled the mental health identity from the very start of the communication, setting the context of acceptability and creating a sense of anxiety and restriction that would be of benefit to the manager in future communications.

These tensions over the access to an illness discourse through which to frame the employee's identity and experience, and the significance of this to the employee, was not only reflected in terminating replies and speech acts, which made clear both the importance and potential severity of the incapacity, but also in the use of certain and potentially inappropriate times in which to conduct these debates. One participant discussed how their manager came to see them at twenty past four on a Friday (the office shut at 4.30 p.m.) in order to tell her that she would not be allowed to apply for a post since they had only just returned from a period of sick leave related to their mental health. With ten minutes remaining on a Friday afternoon, when options for detailed discussion and prolonged negotiation were arguably at their most restrictive, the employee was defined without contest as being unsuitable for promotion due to their sickness identity.

The following case provides a good example of what Kirsch (2000) referred to as the increased stress caused by supervisors in such situations. Here, instead of the establishment of constraints on sickness identity, the employee's manager seeks to construct what is appropriate behaviour once said sickness identity has been embodied; that is, how people with mental ill health should and should not behave. In doing so, this act of constraint represents both a tacit scepticism regarding the legitimacy of the illness and a degree of threat regarding the consequences of moving beyond the acceptable parameters of this construction of illness.

> He said, oh he said I've got a message for you. And he said, oh by the way he said, how are you? And I said not that brilliant C to be honest, I said that's

why I've been signed off. And he said right. I said what's the message? Oh he said, er . . . just to let you know if you decide to shit anywhere in (participant's town) in the next three weeks I will know about it. I said is that it? He said yeah, that's all I wanted to say, and he put the phone down. That was harassment. (Supervisor of a paint shop)

Modes of Identity Negotiation and Discipline

Identities in the context of work have enormous significance because, once fixed, they allow certain ways of relating to and knowing people and so there are processes of discursive labour involved both in this fixing and in resistance whereby the subject, or indeed another actor, has a vested interest in contesting this identity. Deetz (1997) is partly correct that, any control system involves people coming to take the particular subjectivities posited within the system as their own. However, the story in the occupational setting is usually more complex. Identities are more than inevitably constrained elements of control systems that people in some way embody. They are flexible and dynamic entities that individual actors do not passively inhabit but actively manipulate, manoeuvre and utilize in order to contest circumstances arising from their inability to satisfactorily embody traditional worker identities.

In an appraisal of the limitations of Foucault and Butler's notions of subjectivities as dictated by relations of control and dependence, Burkitt (2008) suggests that individuals are not only subject to relations of control but also selves that can be reconstituted within and through their social relations. A good example of this arose with a considerable number of our participants who, when subjective appraisals of their mental health meant that they sought an alleviation of their current circumstances by way of recovery, this action was almost universally met with varying degrees of opposition and sometimes confrontation. The newly formed discursive identity of 'sick individual' had to be used in negotiation in order to assert the need for a process of recovery, a process that was not always felt to be either necessary and/or possible by line managers whose circumstances, needs and requirements were anathema to this identity formation. Knight and Wilmott (1989)'s conception of occupational subjectivities as shifting entities negotiated and constituted through the social practices of organization's was nicely highlighted by our participants' common and sometimes complex use of their newly constructed sickness identities as a bargaining chip with which to secure a degree of authority and influence over their circumstances. Renegotiating appraisals of previously fixed identities inevitably involve the organization bearing new costs in sickness pay and replacement labour for times of sickness. Hence there is a clear motivation behind action to resist and limit the perimeters of effect of these new sickness identities. And so, a process of dialogue often, but not always, ensues where the meaning, scope and consequences of these new identities are disputed in order to achieve Goffman's (1959) agreement on whose claims concerning certain issues will be temporarily honoured.

> The reason why, what happened was that one day I was doing the mail-out and there was some discrepancy about the flyer and there was quite a lot of it left over. Yeah and then he [a director] put me in a spot in front of colleagues and volunteers and one thing I don't like is being grilled and being put on the spot, I don't function well. And when I couldn't come up with any answers as to why there were so many flyers left over he started shouting at me. And he shouted at me, oh yeah, and I said to him, I came back and I said to him 'I think you owe me an apology', and he said 'No I don't!', and he started shouting at me and I think, that's it. The next day I went to my GP and put in a sick note. (Administration Assistant)

It appears that the reason for the immediate consequence of the sickness absence, while possibly linked to feelings of distress following this perceived act of provocation, was partly motivated as a response of empowerment and of retribution as much as self-protection, an act motivated by anger where the sickness identity becomes a possible act of defiance against ill treatment. This complements Wainwright and Calnan's (2002) contention that the work stress discourse is a response to acts of institutional disempowerment, a new mode of labour resistance following the erosion of workplace union and solidarity in recent years. That is not to dismiss the occurrence of physiological and psychological pain due to excessive pressure, rather that there also appears to be a clear link between the embodiment of a specific identity and an act of defiance aimed toward the director. This process of sick role negotiation was often overt rather than an act constructed between employee and GP in the absence of director or managers. In these examples the sick role is used as a way to bargain with a manager.

> I went to my GP and put in a sick note and during that time there was to-ing and fro-ing via email, you know, he wanted me back at work and I wanted

certain conditions met before I would think about work . . . he said 'Oh we need you back, we can't afford to have you sick' and I said to them 'Well, until those conditions are met I'm not coming back and I'm staying off sick. (Administrative Assistant)

The manager's response to the sick note is the suggestion of a return to work which could leave the impression that the sick note does not represent a legitimate response to a genuine illness so much as a break from working. There is no genuine appreciation of the sick role and its ramifications although the overt use of her sickness identity as a resource for bargaining could be taken to reinforce this impression. That said, there is little to suggest that the experience of sickness and the process of using such a sickness identity as a bargaining resource are mutually exclusive, especially where the participant is attempting to secure working conditions that would contribute to her avoiding periods of distress and mental ill health. This process may go some way to influencing Irvine's (2008) finding that line managers found it hard to understand the long term and gradual nature of recovery.

I went and saw my production manager at work, told him I wasn't feeling well. Unless he starts working with me rather than against me and stirring all the shit at work then I will end up going to the doctors and I will be off work. I then saw my big boss, straight out of his office, into his, told him what I told the production manager. (Supervisor of a paint shop)

Well he signed me off with work-related stress and he signed me off for at least a month . . . They wouldn't have a meeting until I came back to work and I said 'No, No I can't go back to work until I've had the meeting because I'm walking back straight into this issue' and then they were going to have one in my home but in the end I decided to go . . . but they said come back to work then we'll have a meeting. They hadn't done anything and I said No, I'm walking straight back into what I left and that . . . and so I said I'm not going to walk back in because I felt as though I was going under. I've never had a breakdown, but I felt very, you know, I was getting terrible pains in my chest, my sleep pattern was bad, you know, because I think it's only work but I was on my own. (Legal Worker)

This participant was keen to have a meeting to negotiate the implications of previous problematic work circumstances that had contributed to his distress and is empowered by the process of having being signed off as sick.

However, here the organization is carefully patrolling the boundaries of what is constructed as an acceptable process for return to work and, as such, directly contributing to the mental distress in the opinion of our participant. This can also be viewed under the auspices of sick role bargaining. The facilitation of a meeting is held to ransom and will be provided only as and when he comes back to work. By definition this act denounces the previously held sickness identity. The identity of illness represents the employee's power to negotiate and to refuse what he considers to be abject treatment. This resonates with Clegg's (1997: p. 29) 'struggle over power' where identities are overtly resisted and fought over.

These processes of negotiation and barter can often take more subtle and implicit forms than the examples above. As with the above example, we have below a reassertion of the organization's power to define the identity and modes of behaviour of employees. Whereas employees who, through mental ill-health, are unable to embody the acceptable discursive constitution of a worker, have at their disposal the considerable identity muscle of the sickness role, representatives of organizations have at their disposal access to possible changes and accommodations in the modes of work that participants are asked to enact. They also have access to information.

The example below differs from above because the assertion of the organizations' will comes not through an explicit instruction or publicly iterated need for more amenable employee behaviour (like coming back to work, rescinding the sick role, attending a meeting on the organization's terms, etc.). Rather, below we have a subtle example where the employer positions themselves as being able to provide information on concerns about the employee's performance, concerns that have been iterated by others. Hence they have access to potentially debilitating constructions of the employee that are occurring in their absence. They concurrently position themselves as being unable to divulge the nature of these performance concerns and implicit in this position is the notion that an early return from sickness, and indeed, the sickness identity, would facilitate the transfer of this information. This rhetorical strategy allows the employer to construct themselves within a discourse of the caring superior, restrained by the rules of both their organization and the inappropriate identity labour of the employee. In this example of identity discipline the 'carrot' is access to these damaging constructions of the sick employee in her absence.

> Some of the things my Manager has said to me over the past year since I've been off sick have been outrageous, such as every time she has a phone call

with me it's 'well actually Marie there have been concerns about your performance'. 'Like what, Julie?' 'I can't tell you that, you're off sick'. (Senior Social Worker)

Yeah, same job, exactly the same job. And when I came back to work I went to see my manager, or my manager asked to see me, and we had a rather strange sort of exchange whereby she sort of said to me '. . . and do you want me to call occupational health?' And it felt like a threat rather than an offer of help. (Administrator)

Another element of subtle coercion mobilized to challenge sickness identity behaviour is exemplified by the occupational health. As with the previous example, the manager is in a position to access a third party. This time, rather than colleagues and their abusive behaviour, it is representatives from occupational health. Occupational Health (OH) is constructed, not as a potential resource for ill workers, but as a body that can be used to instil a degree of discipline and, particularly identity discipline. This quote supports work in the next chapter that outlines OH as a resource for organizations in their battle to ensure that they maintain the balance between public health regulation, potential litigation and employee welfare. In the example above there is no way of knowing whether the comment was intended as a threat, only that in the context of the struggle for apposite identities it was perceived as such. For this individual such a contact meant placing the sickness behaviour on the permanent employee record, an action that at a later date was felt to possibly compromise their employment prospects.

Yes, yes, and so and I just sort of said 'no!' because I didn't know what it meant and I didn't know what the implications were and I thought I might be about to lose my job. (Administrator)

Another example of what Deetz (1997) refers to as 'subtle forms of domination' is provided below. The conflict and uncertainty that often characterize negotiations between employees experiencing mental ill-health and organizations sometimes involve potential discussion over pay. The examples below highlight cases where pay is stopped, or used to come to an arrangement, where the employee with the, by now, troublesome sickness identity is asked to leave should they accept this money. The first example is played through official channels whereas the second example is quite unofficial but both seek to achieve a favourable outcome for the organization at a time where employees are frequently experiencing subjectivities of confusion, guilt and isolation. Indeed the quotes below provide context for Manning and White's (1995) contention that half of employers would never or only occasionally employ someone currently unwell. The first quote below again provides an example of the way that identity disciplining and the struggle to negotiate appropriate worker identities are conducted in the absence of the employee. The organization is constructed as aggressively negotiating for as early a return as possible. Following a period of hospitalization and lack of contact for a single week comes written and contractually justified notification of pay withdrawal. Again the degree of recovery and the duration to which the employee is able to embody the sickness identity is dictated by the financial imperatives of the organization.

> . . . but I thought the Royal Mail managers were actually quite good until recently. They're quite . . . at the moment they're quite sort of . . . when are you coming back? When are you coming back? And quite pushy and I've had a couple of letters saying we're going to stop your pay, because I was in hospital and I hadn't contacted them in the week, because in my contract you've got to contact them . . . (Postman)

> Well it means an awful lot because I had to give up, I was . . . when I had my first illness I had a job working for a charity as a fundraising officer in London, and I, when I returned to work I was offered money like if I left and it was all very unofficial and I felt very badly treated and there was no real care there or anything they just wanted to get rid of me. (Librarian)

Colleagues Reinforcing Identity Discipline: Discourses of Punishment

From the quotes above one might be forgiven for thinking that the contours of identity conflict, negotiation and discipline resemble dichotomous processes where discursive labour is mobilized in order to achieve substantive gains for embattled employees and organizations. However, a number of our participants discussed the way that work colleagues also took on very subtle roles in these processes of disciplining. Kirsh (2000) found that some mental health service users who left their jobs complained that their co-workers treated them differently, once their mental health issue became clear, and there is a detailed body of literature broadly outlining experiences of stigma from colleagues as well as management (Seebohm *et al.*, 2005; Stuart, 2004; Thomas and Secker, 2005; Thornicroft, 2006).

Unlike managers whose dual role as agent of employee welfare and agent of capital accumulation appears to skew irrevocably toward the latter, the participation of colleagues in their mental health experience was only occasionally informed by their conscious awareness and desire to represent the organization. That is, colleagues' participation in these processes of discipline often arose from an intention to act as friend or confidante to the employees who had adopted the sickness identities. The interactions below provide examples of the collective assertion of normality as reinforced through forms of collective censure. Pickering (2001) suggested that it is through censure that normality is defined and legitimate order is maintained. In the work context, legitimate order can represent the personal responsibility of each worker not to be deviant or abnormal in their identity presentation. It is clear from some of the experiences below that colleagues, as well as line managers and directors are implicit in this patrolling of the boundaries between what is legitimate and what is unpalatable to organizations. The presence of a normalizing gaze, the purpose of which is to establish acceptable conduct, involves not only the practices of identity negotiation above but altogether more subtle forms of control that are not direct but are embodied by practices of moral endorsement and enablement (Clegg, 2007). The examples below highlight the way that colleagues transmit practices of discipline that serve, consciously or not, to delegitimize certain sickness identities and behaviours. The conveyance of the manager's anger in the first example serves to create a context of fear, much as might be expected from a more traditional work transgression. By colleagues being enrolled into this unofficial censure and rebuke a culture that is insensitive to future sickness absence possibilities and potential is fostered and reproduced.

> Umm, and then I started to have some time off sick, the odd day here and there. And then I'd had a couple of days off sick and I came in and the guy who I was quite friendly with at work said 'I think you've got to be careful, Jo' – who was my Boss – 'she's been on the war path'. (Administrator)

> She was my Managed Supervisor at the time, I made a complaint about her, because after I went off sick in, the first time in 2000 with panic attacks and everything, she went stomping round the office in a huff, because there was a visit that needed to be done that I therefore wasn't going to do and quite loudly, and all my colleagues told me, she was basically complaining about

the fact that I'd gone off sick and would anyone possibly help do her a favour because – oh, what was it her words were – 'oh I don't suppose you can help your sickly friend out can you and do this visit for her'. (Senior Social Worker)

What I would say is I am aware that one new colleague arrived in something like 2003, Sophie, and she's lovely and we're actually good friends now and she's left as well, but umm, what she said to me was that on her arrival at the office, people had told her to be wary of me, because I'm somebody who is quite needy and needs a lot of support, which I thought was . . . so clearly there was this culture in the office that was sort of 'Marie needs to be . . .' (Senior Social Worker)

In the middle quote a potentially damaging culture of mental health is reproduced through the sardonic use of the work 'sickly'. Moreover an explicit link is formed between the sickness identity and an extra burden of labour for colleagues. Not only do they transmit this anger and in doing so contribute to the process of discipline, they are explicitly recruited as the solution to this inappropriate illness behaviour. Conveying the knowledge of both managerial anger and the consequences of the sickness identity on colleagues' workload is not facilitative of future work absence as a legitimate response to mental ill-health. In the third quote a new colleague reports being recruited into this specific frame of reference regarding the correct and self-protective way of constructing Marie's identity.

In the examples above much of the behaviour is a result of benevolent practices by colleagues aimed either at the employee who has adopted the sickness identity or to new colleagues whose naivety may render them victims of the fallout from the limitations inherent in Marie's deviant employee identity. However, a number of participants reported examples of stigma, abuse, and discrimination and these actions relate to the behaviours above where specific cultures are constructed that legitimate anger, frustration and exclusion as the appropriate responses to sickness identity behaviour. The examples below show that various negative behaviours are constructed as punishment from resentful colleagues to an employee who has adopted the sickness identity. Much of this resentment appears to relate to colleagues' failure to accept the sickness identity as legitimate and hence not warranting either a short or prolonged period away from the workplace. The suffering and subjective distress appears to be configured in the terms of how it affects the colleagues in terms of workload. There appears to have been a collective decision taken to construct the absent employee as someone who has control over the degree to which they feel distress and hence the participant as 'selfish' for this prolonged absence. Colleagues also had clear boundaries regarding what was acceptable sickness behaviour and, while these are not explicitly stipulated, his worker's absence of seven months from work clearly conflicts with these:

> Well they were very resentful for the time I had off. It didn't seem to occur to them that I might have a genuine reason for being off. I went off on the seventeenth of September so they were just very annoyed because it made Christmas more stressful for them at work and socially. And they said 'oh that was wrong of me, selfish of me', and they couldn't understand why I'd need to be off seven months and I mean eventually I did sort of like ask one of them why they weren't speaking, why they weren't speaking to me and this is kind of what their explanation was. (Cook in a residential home)

> I decided when I went back to work 'I'll look for another job', . . . my relationship with them had broken down and I wasn't, I was on the look-out for another job. And you know, I went in as normal, and I know because my relationship with them was very difficult and very cold and I couldn't give a toss what they thought or think, that was none of my concern. (Administration Assistant)

> There was three original people . . . ganging up really, stirring up of one of the people . . . to complain about me and it was soon after that the problem started. . . . When I went off sick they were okay, you know, it was tolerable but then when I went back off of being off sick, they didn't speak to me for a month. (Cook in a residential home)

> . . . (I would) only come on the condition that I have somebody coming in with me an advocate because I couldn't trust my colleagues; it was such a small company. (Administration Assistant)

Returns to work were characterized in some cases not so much by aggressive or punishing or disciplining actions but by a lack of awareness over how to behave in these hugely unconventional situations. However, a considerable number of the experiences of people returning to work were characterized by conflict and tension. This resonates with Eakin's (2005) discourse of abuse where workplaces were often characterized by embedded expectations that those in the work injury support system were typically party to a violation of its entitlements. Stuart (2004) notes that when many mental health service users return to work they often do so in positions of reduced responsibility and with little or no psychosocial support from colleagues. While this is undoubtedly the case, it fails to really capture the full implications of the social practices that people experience on return to work from both short and long absences. The discourses of abuse and punishment and the dramaturgical cooperation (Goffman, 1959) either consciously or unconsciously between the colleagues and management which so often characterizes these social responses to sick employees have the effect of legitimizing a culture where mental ill-health is the responsibility of, and under the control of, employees. Employees who fall foul of this maxim face social sanctions.

In some cases the proliferation of normalizing gazes can reproduce managerial frustration with sickness absences and in others cooperate in the expression of moral sanctions for inappropriate sickness/employee identity. To a degree, this reflects Deetz's (1992: p. 40) claim that 'no management group can control the actions, let alone the thoughts of other groups. The presence of fear (warranted or not), assumptions of knowledge differences . . . must be provided by the controlled groups'.

The (Re)Construction of The Substandard Employee

This final and complimentary process, fundamental to the negotiation of sickness identities, concerns appraising and reappraising the work performances of the sick employees either in their presence, absence or return to work. Very often there is a rhetorical reconstruction of absent employees that embodies Clegg's (2007) assertion that identities in the work place are not absolute but always relational. Frequently, employees who experience poor mental health, tend to adhere to the 'good employee' discourse. That is, employees play the role of continuing to show a willingness to commit to the organization while engaging in some form or stress management or psychotherapeutic intervention that moves them toward recovery. Implicit in this is what Harkness et al. (2005) call the unwritten rule of 'be happy or else'. This section shows that the 'or else' can take the form of management drawing upon a discourse of substandard employee performance in order to constitute or, more often, reconstitute the work history of sick employees as always having been somehow inherently problematic, even before the period of mental ill health. This practice often represents a reformulation of the employees' history that moves beyond the processes of discipline and punishment above toward a rhetoric that lays the groundwork for procedures that allow the organization to move toward dismissal. In this way, economic interests are protected against the threat of prolonged sickness pay, and temporary replacement employees. Occasionally, but not always, it is a practice enacted following failed attempts to negotiate an employee sickness identity that is satisfactory to the imperatives of management and represents the establishment of control over a situation by (re) defining the situation (Goffman, 1959).

> ... by the time this meeting came I was actually fed up. I'd had a major complaint lodged against me, which was so totally unfounded that even a child could have seen that it was trumped up and they were messing around. They hadn't responded to his letter for 3 months, you know, if you wrote a letter of complaint, wouldn't you be a bit miffed if they hadn't even said thank you for your letter. (Laughs) ... but there was no apology when they found there was no case to answer. By this time I was off sick because I couldn't cope with it. (Legal Worker)

> I had a particularly difficult meeting with my Manager, again this was about 2004, in which she basically said that she was going to take me to an investigative meeting because someone had told her that I'd left a case file in the boot of my car. And I had a panic attack and then she said to me 'do you need an asthma pump?' I said 'I'm not asthmatic Julia, I'm having a panic attack! [Laughs]' (Administration Assistant)

For the purposes of this analysis we have no way of corroborating the veracity of the complaint but the fact that the legal worker above interpreted it as such represented at the very least a monumental breakdown of communication and trust and at the most a cynical attempt to duplicitously remove an employee on what were potentially unreasonable grounds. In the above case it appeared that a colleague's suspicion of the participant's unprofessional behaviour was sufficient grounds for the launch of an investigation, an action that was precipitated before the incident was verified with the participant. The participant was unsure that this transition to an investigative meeting would have occurred had there not already been suspicions regarding her competence on the grounds of her mental ill health.

In the case below, faced with the altogether more challenging task of addressing mental health, the employer sought refuge in unwarranted disciplinary procedures which the sick employee barely had the resources to defend.

> On the 6th July last year I was due to go back to work (following being off work with clinical depression), and went along to what I thought was going to be a return to work interview, when my Manager suddenly told me that she'd done an investigation, and accused me of fabricating information and case conference reports – I'm a Senior Social Worker in Child Protection – umm, and told me that they were going to take me through formal capability procedures at stage three, which ultimately meant that it could lead to dismissal or redeployment and what she was recommending was that I be redeployed outside of xxx Child Care Social Work. (Senior Social Worker)

This employee talked about how she went from a senior worker, of 14 year's experience, who many other workers used to seek out for help and guidance on such activity as preparing court statements, to someone who had 'never really been able to do her job' as a result of, in her opinion, her period of mental ill health. The case below highlights a worker who, although much earlier in her period of employment than the participant above, and following a period of struggling with ill health, was told that she was causing problems due to her not doing her work properly. Once her sickness identity had been rejected and supplanted by a work performance discourse the atmosphere became very strained and indeed contributed to her need to seek help.

> My Manager's approach with me was 'you're causing problems for everyone else because you're not doing the work properly' so there was an awareness of, I suppose I was thinking well, you know, I'm sort of being labelled as this person who's causing all these problems because I'm not working hard enough and it was that undercurrent of knowing that people were aware of that, or had been told that and yet were being kind of nice to my face – I suppose they weren't bad people'. (Administrator)

> Umm, so, we had this meeting and we agreed that – I mean what I didn't want was for, to be given, I was still in my probationary period, what I didn't want was just to suddenly be given a two-week notice which I could have been given – so we arranged I think for six weeks notice to try and get me another job, so that I would have time to get another job. I went in for a few days, but the atmosphere was really difficult and so after a few days I went to see my Doctor and . . . (Administrator)

Another participant reported that her manager, despite being legally obliged, wasn't prepared to discuss any adjustments to her job. In being told that she was 'not doing the work, you're going to have to find another job' she found her previous good working relationship reformulated as always having being intermittently problematic, although the participant could not recall any informal or official record of this new problematic work history. One employee talked about how her manager confronted her to tell her that she had had 'concerns about her performance for two months' following which she went into a long list of tasks that the employee was unable to do. This manager, knowing that the employee had a prior history of depression, had been advised by occupational health that the employee should receive additional management support. However, this litany of employment errors and imperfections had been stored for two months as evidence of the employee's performance and it was through a discourse of poor work performance that these events were reconstructed with no mention of potential mental ill health as a source.

One of our participants noted how she 'was called in to have a meeting' upon which her manager was 'really quite aggressive'. This process of unexpectedly being called into a meeting to be confronted with a litany of work performance complaints, examples of failure to meet work standards or prolonged observations of ineptitude and struggle and occasionally aggression and intransigence, were not uncommon. Sometimes it occurred even in conditions where line managers had been advised to or had agreed to have regular meetings or adjustments but which had failed to materialize. And this process frequently caught employees off-guard. They had little or no preparation or knowledge of the litany of complaints that had left previously satisfied managers convinced of their need to find another job. Indeed it was frequently interpreted as pre-planned preparation for a meeting that had at its core the single goal of convincing the employee, through recollection of their manifested incompetencies, that they had to leave. It would not be an unnecessarily sensationalist metaphor to suggest that these encounters took on the sense of a pre-planned ambush. Unprepared, unaided, alone and often low of confidence, clarity and energy if they were experiencing mental ill health at the time, employees did not always have the resources to effectively resist these disputed charges. For those participants drawn from the employment and mental health project, these experiences preceded their involvement with the organization.

The participant below, following dismissal by the company, outlines how it might be possible that his employers had acted upon potentially problematic events that were not only constructed as part of the job but that counteracted his own knowledge and history as a good employee. Self-confidence for employees during times of mental ill health is typically low (Cameron et al., 2010, Under Review) and despite this knowledge he did not have sufficient confidence to resist the circumstances of his termination.

> It was because they didn't think I was good at my job and I thought well I know I am, a couple of people complained but then people do complain because in anything now, consumer related, people have such high standards and they can be quite unreasonable and if you don't jump; . . . I just felt less confident in dealing with my own one-to-one's with people. . . . Clients would ring up and say 'oh thank you so much'. (Legal Worker)

Refusing to grant a colleague or employee a sickness identity, or supplanting this with an identity based on substandard work performance, is potentially facilitative of a number of employer goals. Firstly, it allows companies to construct what would be a potentially problematic and financially costly and unpredictable employee as beyond saving. It makes inevitable their need to move toward dismissal for the good of the organization and other employees and indeed the problem employee themselves. If their problem is based on an inability to perform the job then dismissal can be presented as an act of charity. Constructing the person experiencing mental ill health as a substandard employee, and with little attention to Disability Discrimination Act requirements, allows a diminution of guilt and personal culpability on the part of managers who are often under pressure to meet productivity targets. It is also beneficial to colleagues who are inconvenienced directly by the extra workload that comes with sickness absence. Rather than as a friend and colleague who requires support in a time of need, they become a colleague who perpetually lets others down with their lack of aptitude or engagement with the tasks of the job. Such constructions, especially of an employee who is relatively new to the organization, have clear benefits and may have contributed to the actions above. Moreover it is possible that in the cultures of increasing work intensity (Purcell et al., 1999; European Foundation for the Improvement of Living and Working Conditions, 2000; Lapido and Wilkinson, 2002; Burchell, 2002; Taylor et al., 2003; Coffey and Dugdill, 2006) outlined in chapter 1, the pressure to construct these substandard identities has increased in recent years.

Conclusion

> . . . and feeling that all my energy was going into defending myself. All my energy was going into worrying about being attacked and being portrayed

in a very negative way and that all my energy was going into worrying about that and thinking about how I would fend that off. (Administrator)

The central message that comes from this chapter is not whether medical discourses are or are not in any absolute sense the most appropriate way to understand periods of mental suffering in and around work. Nor does it provide an appraisal of the employment and mental health service used by the participants since the processes outlined in this chapter occurred before the use of this service. Rather it is to explore how these discourses and others are drawn upon by different actors in different circumstances and to fulfil different obligations. Having access to a medical discourse with which to present your employee identity, and hence to periods and practices of illness recuperation, is not automatic. In many cases this access is tightly circumscribed by social relationships and practices that fulfil organizational and in some cases personal imperatives. Gorz (1999) noted that little physical or psychical space remained which is not occupied by the company, what he defined as the 'opposite of a free subjectivity'. The conflicts above evidence resistance, constraint and negotiation over the way that people are able to present themselves. Employee identities that fail to reflect organizational logic are deviant and represent a threat to the accumulation of capital. They fail to embody the deliberative, universally adaptive and self-regulating subjects so complimentary to neoliberal capital accumulation (Walkerdine, 2002) and are punished for this transgression. This still appears to be the case despite considerable recent progress with disability discrimination legislation. Our work supports Baldamus's view of industrial relations as 'a structure of differentiated power that reflects unequally distributed advantages and disadvantages' (Baldamus, 1961: p. 7).

The conflicts above regarding the way that people are able to perform their illnesses and the consequences of these performances exist at the juncture of a number of competing and in some cases diametrically opposed interests. The formal and informal practices of control and discipline enacted by a number of managers reflect Wainwright and Calnan's (2002) notion of capital's retaliation against increasingly prohibitive and restrictive health and safety legislation, itself an individualized manifestation of worker empowerment following the recent diminution of organized labour solidarity.

In this chapter we considered problematic constructions of adjustments, processes of controlling the sick role, modes of identity negotiation and discipline, discourses of punishment and the selective reproduction of the sick employee through discourses of employee incompetence. Reflecting on these practices it becomes clear that there are interesting parallels with Reid et al.'s (1991) work with sufferers of repetitive strain injury (RSI) at work. As with mental health, sufferers of RSI are required to disabuse notions of health incapacitation as a channel to employee delinquency. The condition has an uncertain aetiology and there are public and private questions over its very legitimacy as a valid medical entity. Reid noted that the political meaning of RSI was rooted in capitalist labour processes exemplified by the concomitant and seemingly infinite search for greater control over workers and greater efficiency of their work. We would contend that the way that we understand and perform mental health is also intimately rooted in these capitalist labour processes of control and this chapter represents an attempt to illustrate how these control processes are both made manifest and resisted. Sickness identities are direct confrontations to the control of labour, and the occasional brutality of capitals' foot soldiers should be taken as the result of line managers and colleagues being inevitably and forcefully thrust into subjectivities that patrol the work identities of those around them; as the often unwilling agents and victims of the domineering rationalist logic of Anglo-American capitalism. When Black (2008) notes that as many as 40% of organizations have no sickness absence management policy, one should be very clear that this does not mean that so many organizations do not have culturally and economically proscribed practices of sickness absence management.

To understand, as Jackson and Carter (1997) have suggested, the way that techniques of power are invented to meet the demands of production, it is necessary to draw upon both symbolic and materialist perspectives that suggest the work of Gorz and Foucault. Potential mental health experiences are refracted through modern capital's permitted and domineering practices of identity negotiation, conflict and discipline. As such, one might expect that recent and well documented increases in work intensity (Burchell, 2002; Coffey and Dugdill, 2006; European Foundation for the Improvement of Living and Working Conditions, 2000; Lapido and Wilkinson, 2002; Purcell et al., 1999; Taylor et al., 2003) will potentially exacerbate these problematic social practices. Recent neoliberal structural changes in the UK have led to a diminution of workplace protections, the erosion of solidarity and an increasing intensity of work for a growing number of people. In this framework it becomes easier to empathize with overworked employees whose perception of a colleagues' ill-health translates not in social, human or empathic terms but as a representation of extra workload. Moreover it is an extra workload that they are forced to shoulder in a time of diminishing labour capacities and executive logic that outlaws expensive replacements.

There are an increasing number of people looking for employment in neoliberal political cultures where the rationale of efficiency savings, bolstered by an increasingly expeditious technology sector, has made an increasing number of people surplus to requirements (Gorz, 1999). It may well be the case that the combination of these social, political, economic and historical events decreases the potential of employees experiencing mental ill health to resist these rhetorical practices of discipline and oppressive identity management. In this context one might suggest that any understanding of line managers as being able to fulfil the dual roles of agent of capital, via practices of marshalling productivity, and agent of their employee's well-being is at best wildly optimistic.

Far from representing an exhaustive list of the social practices of negotiation that occur during mental ill health at work, this chapter attempts to provide a snapshot that frames some of these experiences and thus act as a counterpoint to the individualistic and atomizing ideological fervour of mainstream psychological literature and policy that frames mental health at work as an employee issue. To understand cultures of work it is necessary to understand the way that political and economic practices impact on people both objectively and through their subjective comprehension of material and rhetorical processes of marginalization and resistance. It is insufficient and indeed complimentary to neoliberal political rationalities to simply isolate and seek to 'put right' the resulting subjectivities of suffering through therapy and stress reduction techniques. This work allows us to reject any precept that posits an understanding of experiences of mental ill health at work as resulting from a series of internal cognitive attributes. Any approach that seeks to ameliorate and 'recover' an employee with a view to return to work cannot ignore these practices of discrimination, discipline and identity negotiation that are central to the experience of suffering at work. A recent report by the UK office of the Deputy Prime Minister (2004) suggested that early sensitive and regular contact with employees during sickness absence could be a key factor in early return to work. This chapter outlines the possibility that such contact, for many workplaces, is far from straightforward and indeed may militate directly against such potentially positive outcomes.

Chapter 5

Managing Mental Health in Organizations

The previous chapter attempted to provide an account of the ways in which some people can experience the negotiation of sickness identities in modern workplaces. In doing so we provided an analysis that framed the performance and experience of mental ill health as intimately and inevitably rooted in capitalist labour processes. It is our contention that without understanding these processes of control and identity negotiation, and the economic pressures by which they are driven, it is not possible to effectively formulate a theory of practice that seeks to address the discriminating and marginalizing processes that occur in many UK workplaces. Socially mediated practices where sickness identities are defended, reproduced, negated and contested, embody the logic of modern neoliberal capital accumulation. In providing this account it does not represent a formidable task to construct the principal actors through pantomime representations of villainy and foul play. The point of the previous chapter was never to denigrate one specific group of organization actors as in some way 'responsible' for converting the capitalist labour logic into interpersonal terms of abuse, exploitation and cruelty. Rather it is our contention that modern organizations function as social machines or social control systems whereby the elaborate discourses of information and knowledge that dictate potential identities, and the 'tactics of power' (McKinlay and Starkey, 1997) inherent in these forms of discourse, frame line manager and supervisor subjectivities that are exceptionally difficult to resist.

That is not to say that there are no sites for resistance. Rather, it is to say that, to a large extent, the line managers in many UK organizations are

Work and the Mental Health Crisis in Britain, First Edition. C. Walker and B. Fincham.
© 2011 John Wiley & Sons, Ltd. Published 2011 by John Wiley & Sons, Ltd.

subject to the same practices of moral endorsement and enablement that they themselves enact upon their staff. While decision making latitude is a privilege for many managers it should be noted that, far from being self-governing agents of oppression and tyranny, they themselves come to inhabit relatively fixed identities that permit certain ways of relating to staff and certain ways of knowing the organization. In the shareholder brand of capitalism they exist in a system whereby productivity and the delivery of improving profit margins serve to dictate the degree to which subjectivities of benevolence, empathy and flexibility are enacted. This mode of capitalism is evident in the UK and, as opposed to state-led or consensual/stakeholder modes of capitalism (Schmidt and Hersh, 2006), managers have the primary duty to maximize shareholder results (Smith, 2003). Should they fail to deliver this outcome, through mental ill health, compassion or empathy then they themselves fall under scrutinizing and disciplinary gazes, the very same practices of endorsement and enablement.

It is for this reason that line managers, the actors so intimately involved in the administration of the practices of discipline and tactics of power discussed in the previous chapter, should be seen as subject to the same control systems as employees. It is in an uneasy and contradictory position that many line managers come to find themselves; that is, the arbiters of productivity-based discipline and the institutionally sanctioned providers of employee support against the ramifications of some of these very practices of productivity.

This chapter seeks to explore this potential contradiction and the tensions and difficulties that many line managers, and indeed more senior managers, experience in the face of competing role dynamics. Thirty managers were drawn from organizations in the South East of England in order to take part in interviews regarding mental health and work. They were drawn from public, private and voluntary sector organizations and were asked about a number of issues related to mental health at work. The majority of managers were line managers managing small teams although a number of senior managers were also interviewed from these three sectors. This chapter will outline the ways in which managers in the UK today act as capable and skilled conduits of various government and organization policies on mental ill health. We will explore whether managers have experienced the postulated increases in employee work intensity and indeed whether neoliberal modes of profit enhancement have changed the working experiences of line managers and their staff. Moreover, we will look at managerial reflections on the processes of discrimination, harassment and marginalization prevalent in a growing literature (Eakin, 2005; Office of the Deputy Prime Minister, 2004; Stuart, 2004; Thomas and Secker, 2005; Thornicroft, 2006).

Mental Health Policy and Practice: The Managerial Experience

Much of the research literature on experiences of mental ill health and work suggests that if you spend time looking for experiences of discrimination and stigma then you will invariably find them (Eakin, 2005; Office of the Seebohm 2005; Stuart, 2004; Thomas and Secker; 2005; Thornicroft, 2006). However much of this work focuses on the working lives of the employees who, due to their experiences of mental ill health and associated absences from work, have found themselves at the mercy of work cultures that often lack both empathy and accommodation. Less ubiquitous are accounts from the managers who find themselves enforcing, arbitrating, defending and moderating institutionally inscribed modes of practice.

Stuart (2004) states that over 50% of employers expressed discomfort at hiring someone with a previous mental health hospitalization. In the US, 33% of mental health consumers (Stuart's terminology) have been turned down for a job contingent on their disclosure of histories of mental ill health, 78% of mental health service users in Bristol reported having lost one or more jobs as a result of mental illness and between a third and a half were dismissed, were forced to resign or were made redundant due to discrimination (Thomas and Secker, 2005). Moreover, 47% of mental health service users described experiences of often incredibly painful discrimination at work (Thornicroft, 2006). Therefore, one might expect that the recent UK Department of Health initiative to improve mental health in the workplace via the amelioration of stigma (Shift, 2007) might be hamstrung by ambitious terms of reference. The principles of the campaign concern the promotion of 'a culture of respect and dignity for everyone' and to encourage the awareness of mental health issues. 89% of managers agreed with the laudable egalitarian principles of the campaign. The problem of course is a potential void between beliefs and practice. Since only 25% of managers were thought to be aware of the procedures in their organization for addressing mental health problems (Shift, 2007), perhaps this void is predicated on ignorance and inadequate mental health training?

If managers are expected to satisfactorily manage employee mental ill health then one might firstly ask why so many managers remain ignorant of procedures. More importantly, does it really matter?

The principle reason that this question is so important is because the UK Health and Safety Commission's Health and Safety Executive (HSE) relies on managerial knowledge and motivation to implement their management standards to reduce the growing problem of work-related stress in British workers (The Health and Safety Executive, 2005). The HSE desires that employers work with employees to implement stress management standards, in order to work to reduce the growing number of people who have experienced work-related stress, at a level that they believe has made them ill. Through the regulation and provision of supporting relationships, managing change, consultation and employee empowerment, employers (and this is, in practice, very often line managers) have a duty (although not compulsorily enforced) to ensure that risks arising from work are properly controlled. Indeed with specific relevance to stigma, systems should be in place such that people are able to respond to individual concerns lest there be bullying and discrimination. The Trades Union Congress welcomed the standards and noted that in the absence of legislation the HSE guidelines were the most effective tool that employers could use to help end what they referred to as an 'epidemic of stress related illnesses' (The Health and Safety Executive, 2005).

In 2005, the UK government reiterated their awareness of stress as a significant contributing factor to sickness leave and noted that the HSE is addressing this through the management standards approach (HM Government, 2005). The first part of this chapter highlights the challenges and contradictions that characterize the day to day working experiences of many managers. We then investigate the ways in which line managers experience, respect and ultimately reproduce the policies and employment guidance that have been generated by the government and/or by their employers.

Line Managers – Challenges and Contradictions

A primary component of managing workers in Britain in the twenty-first century for many people is the tension between what we might perhaps call a human reaction to responsibilities at work and a more instrumental reaction to responsibilities at work. This is best summed up by the conflict some managers feel between the 'duty of care' they have to staff beneath them versus their obligations to the productivity of the employing organization. This tension has increased over time as working practices have been [and are] subject to regimes of intensification, job insecurity,[1] 'lean' productive techniques and a perceived decline in job discretion (Burchell et al., 2002; Gorz 1999; Green, 2004). For us there are attendant issues of health that arise from the working situations prone to these changes over time. Firstly problems with work are understood to be residing in the individual worker – and manifest themselves as health issues. Secondly, workers tend to be managed on the whole by line managers who, practically, have little scope to bring about meaningful changes in the work organization of employees – necessary for the alleviation of problems – and who are themselves struggling with similar problems. Thirdly, these problems are often managed largely by people with relatively poor mental health literacy – given the responsibility they actually have for people's well-being – and are largely unsupported by their senior management or directors.

For many of our managers the responsibility thrust upon them by their position in a hierarchy led to particular concerns about responsibility. Were they responsible to those beneath them in the hierarchy or to those above? As has been discussed in the sections on policies there is an expectation that troubling aspects of managing others, particularly if they become unwell, can be militated against with the utilization of robust or clear procedures and structures. Whilst this might be the perception it does not appear to match the experiences of the people that we spoke to.

For the purposes of illustration this next section is organized between discussing *duty of care* – the terrain where the concerns of individual managers about individual colleagues and health are played out – and *obligations to productivity* – the terrain where managers are tasked with pursuing corporate objectives. It is also where managers are managed and their instrumental function comes into conflict with the relationships they have with those they manage. In the section on *obligations to productivity* there are specific discussions on managers as managed and the implications of sick leave for line managers. These discussions are presented as examples of the conflicted role line managers routinely face within their instrumental role – that is to say – as employees they are in a formal hierarchy and with sick leave they are invoking a formal process.

---

[1] As opposed to job stability.

Duty of Care

There is a large literature addressing issues of managerial styles (see for example Benfari 1991; Bjerke, 2001; Bass *et al.*, 1975; Ladegaard, 2011; Rees, 1996; Weightman, 1999) and in particular workplace relationships that extend 'beyond the formal obligations of the employment contract' (Wainwright and Calnan, 2002, p. 110). The thrust of much of this literature is that the informal social relations that can form in workplaces promote sets of quasi familial bonds that are good for people working together.[2] Related to this there is a literature on what is known as the 'ethical climate' – suggesting that organizations have an ethical responsibility to foster relations predicated on shared understandings between owners, senior managers or board members and employees (Armstrong and Francis, 2008; Martin and Cullen, 2006). This literature, focused more on leadership responsibility and is more hierarchical in its approach, and more importantly, is predicated on the idea that individuals in organizations operate within ethical parameters established at an institutional level. Whilst not refuting such observations altogether, the data gathered in the mental health and work study that we conducted suggested something more akin to traditional hierarchy, still human and personal – but the moral or ethical parameters are established at an individual level. Managers, on the whole, felt a duty of care to those below them in the hierarchy, and would often attempt to adapt working practice, protest or subvert institutional expectations in order to protect or support their colleagues on lower scales. This often involved more work for them. It was frequently the case that a combination of institutional responsibility combined with a sense of personal responsibility drove the actions of managers to staff and particularly to those that had become unwell. Some spoke in a very general way about their relationship to those below them in the hierarchy:

> I always feel that my staff are my staff and I protect them; even if I do have to tell them off behind closed doors. (Senior Retail Manager)

Others referred to specific incidents. One private sector manager recalled her reaction to a particular employee that was struggling:

---

[2] It is interesting to note that this language is the same as used by Gorz when describing the debilitating effects of subjection that we referred to earlier in chapter 1.

... [colleagues had] seen him just sitting at the bar, as somebody put it, 'like a little old man just getting drunk;' he was only twenty two or three, and eventually I managed to coax him into the office and speak to him. The funny thing there was that I felt really torn between being an employer and being old enough to be his mother almost. (Recruitment Consultancy Manager)

She then went on to describe how she tried to reintegrate him into a team that was suspicious of his condition. Whilst the language used by this manager fits with the familial analogy, her drawing on a maternal metaphor suggests something less instrumental than 'we are all in this together' implied by a corporate 'family'. It is something altogether more human and less abstract. Another manager in the private sector talked about her dealing with a young man who suffered with depression that she was managing:

Because none of the rest of the staff knew what was going on and they were partly puzzled by me, because I am quite a determined manager and one of my abilities is to increase productivity in people but ... so they were a bit surprised I think that I wasn't leaping up and down in the back saying 'why aren't you doing things?' and it's because I realized, I watched him and I thought this isn't right. (Senior Retail Manager interview)

In this instance there is a tacit expectation that the role of the manager is to be punitive in dealing with transgression, irrespective of the reasons behind such behaviour. Once again the human reaction to the situation overtook the rational, instrumental worth of the employee. This manager was relating to another person who was struggling.

This was expressed by another manager but the response, whilst clearly causing some internal conflict followed the formal strictures of managerial responsibilities to the workplace and not the worker:

... and that was really difficult because the more pressure I was putting on her was making her unwell, and then she did go off and she went off for about seven months in the end with stress and depression. And then she kind of came back and that was very difficult because you feel in a very torn position 'cos you know, she has suicidal thoughts and everything, and to supervise somebody is just going way out of the work area, it's all about her own life and that, knowing that she was very lonely and depressed and knowing what I was doing, even though I had to do what I needed to do, that was actually making her unwell, and it was my job to actually get people into work! (Supported Employment Manager for a housing association)

In terms of developing strategies that would appear to undermine the corporate objectives of intensification of work, one manager spoke about a strategy she has developed to militate against people working too many hours.

> I mean if I'm in the office I'll have spotted they're there too late and say 'you probably should have gone by now.' I will surreptitiously give each of them some time back if I see it happening enough. (Senior Retail Manager)

A cynical view of this could be that it is not in the interests of the organization, or of those managing within them to have a workforce that is overstretched and overtired. However, as has been seen elsewhere, this is the common experience of work as reported to us.

Another manager in the voluntary sector recounted an experience that she had with an employee whose mental health condition had led to an encounter with the police, which was subsequently logged on a Criminal Records Bureau (CRB) check:

> We have a human resources department based in our office in London. They got the results of the CRB check and said 'right we are going to have to suspend her immediately'... I then interviewed her as her line manager with somebody from HR with me and asked her just to explain about this incident, just to get her version of things and she was great. She was absolutely open and honest, you know and very cooperative. It must have been really difficult for her. (Social Work Manager)

This particular manager, whilst following organizational procedures, felt particularly protective of somebody that she described as 'great' at work. What later transpired is that the manager was in the process of developing strategies that would mean the employee could remain at work and that the human resources department were satisfied that the organization would not be compromised by the continued employment of this particular person.

This was a common theme amongst the managers that we spoke to. Many reported that they became responsible for designing ways of working that would enable people that the employing organization would in the normal course of things replace. Such managers responded to their personal feelings of obligation to those they were managing despite the easiest option might have been to bow to the institutional pressure for optimum productivity.

The tension created between day to day responsibilities for the well-being of those that line managers manage appears to be a source of particular anxiety for many. Several people spoke about this in relation to the outsourcing of personnel or human relations departments. One manager in the civil service explained that the nature of the outsourced 'support' meant that one person that needed an intervention had to travel a significant distance, to another county, to be assessed by people they did not know. The implementation of a strategy designed by occupational health then became the sole responsibility of the manager in the workplace. Whilst this might not sound dissimilar to a more traditional model of occupational health support, the fact that the support network was not 'in house' created particular problems of timing and contactability.

Obligation to Productivity

The human reaction to the problems of others is balanced for many by the demands of their responsibilities to the organizations that employ them. As has been suggested it is the tension between wanting to do the best for those that are managed and wanting to meet the corporate objectives of their various organizations and businesses that appears to be a particular concern for many of the people that we interviewed:

> I think it is around pressure points, it's around when there are deliverables that impact down the line. (University Manager)

As with much else in discussion about intensity of work, this process was characterized as increasing incrementally:

> Companies set these goals and they are impossible to meet. (Former Public Relations Manager)

> Within this organization there is a culture around, you know, I mean I've got a Blackberry, all the senior managers have got Blackberrys, and there is a culture that on Sunday evening people are e-mailing . . . I think what we've done is we've adopted the corporate way of working which is actually that, you know, nothing can wait. (Senior Executive in Mental Health Trust)

> Suddenly we've all got targets and budgets, but what does it mean and there's people going 'well I wasn't trained to do any of this'. (University Dean of Faculty)

In an interview with a senior manager in a retail business the conflict between economic rationalism and the tendency to want to do the best for people was made clear. This conflict was played out between the interviewee and her seniors in the organization:

> People who actually own the business, because I was running the business, said just, you know, 'get rid of him'. I said 'you can't do that'. (Senior Retail Manager)

Later in the same passage she described how she tried to appeal to the better nature of the owners by saying 'he's a nice guy, he's not doing this on purpose, he doesn't know how to control it' (Senior Retail Manager). The perception that middle managers are buffers between the workers and the malign intentions of senior managers was common and was reflected throughout our interviews. This is expanded upon later in the chapter.

When asked about the incentive for a large organization for developing ways of working that might benefit those who were struggling with mental health problems one manager in the voluntary sector said:

> There would be no room for it . . . absolutely not because it's, you know, outcomes drive. It's task driven, it's, you know, that concept that you create work around the strengths of the individual is anti many management models. (Children's Charity Manager)

The conflict was clearly expressed at an abstract level, and people were subsequently able to identify areas where the tension between their emotional attachment or their social responsibility to employees ran up against the corporate productive logic of their own employers. Two interesting areas that were spoken about were the sense of managers themselves being managed – or not – and then the issue of managing sick leave. We have chosen to briefly discuss these two areas because they appear to raise distinct concerns, but are connected in the way they position middle managers in relation to productive processes that do not match with personal concerns about the well-being of themselves or, in the case of sick leave, others.

Example 1: Managers Managed

The capacity that managers feel they have to change whole systems is curtailed by their own position as employees. This enforces the Gorzian view that: 'autonomy' within parameters established by somebody else is no sort of autonomy, and a feature of the position of managers is their perception of themselves as being managed by others. As we have mentioned, many of the people that we spoke to saw themselves as being caught between two sets of interests – those of the people they were managing and those that managed them. It is also the case that, as with the discussion about long working hours, there is a myth about the positive aspects of increased autonomy. It appears that 'autonomy' is for many shorthand for an increase of individualized working. In this respect 'autonomy' becomes 'sense of responsibility' towards both employers and employees. This middle ground is a particularly difficult place to occupy, where expectations of performance are measured outside of contractual obligations – like long working hours, working from home, making sure that everybody's well-being is being satisfactorily protected. Several people talked about this ambiguous position as one of isolation:

> Managers are much more isolated and that's more difficult either to tell the person above you, or because you're managing other people to not reflect that downwards, so where do I go, or where do [others at a similar grade] go in that situation? (University Manager)

The sense that they are accountable to a variety of people with differing interests was also a key determinant in managers' feelings of isolation. Having explained the responsibility they felt towards their staff, two managers then talked about wider corporate expectations and their impact on their work in different ways. One spoke about direct expectations of his former manager:

> At my last job which I was at for three years ... if you were coming in at 9 and going home at 5.30 then the boss would be thinking, you know, 'where's the extra effort'? (Line Manager in communications firm)

The other spoke about to whom he felt accountable. Rather than being responsive in two directions – those above him and those below him, he said:

> A lot more than two directions, blimey. Got the trustees to look after who are the people who are actually financially liable for the organization, you know all the decisions I make wouldn't come back to me in court, they'd come back to my employers. Every registered charity has to have a board of

trustees and directors who are financially and legally liable. (Community Development Manager)

There is a broader sense of corporate responsibility being shouldered by this manager in as much as he has a sense of a diverse structure operating above him to which he is accountable but with whom he has little interaction.

Much of what we were told by managers relates to corporate expectations of autonomous working. For many this autonomy is experienced as being cut adrift from any formal management that might provide the sorts of structures they feel it necessary to provide for those they manage. This in conjunction with intensification of working practice, impacts on well-being. The tension is then turned towards responsibility to the self versus productive responsibilities. As a brand manager at a distribution firm said of other managers:

> It's affecting their mental health. It's bringing stress to them, and I have encountered many people that have been signed off work through stress from work and have got better at home and have come back to work. I myself have been fairly close to just, you know, just jacking in the job and saying 'fuck you' and walking off. (Brand Manager in distribution firm)

Example 2: Coping with/Implications of Sick Leave

A problem many of the managers described was the responsibility they felt when managing sick leave. It is at this point that the instrumental corporate identity often superseded the more humanistic pastoral identity. The corporate environment was not geared for treating certain problems sympathetically. As one respondent said:

> It's certainly not respected in our organization, people going off with stress. (Children's charity Manager).

Having said this most of the managers still struggled with the balance that they had to strike between productivity, for which they were partly responsible, on the one hand, and the well-being of those below them in a hierarchy on the other. One manager talked of the difficulty caused when somebody does not disclose problems that they are having:

> Quite often people will keep things from you, they don't want you to know and that's really hard because when something has completely collapsed you're then asked to try and pick up the pieces and that's actually quite painful for everybody including the people who are trying to hide it from you and getting people to learn from that experience is really hard. (University Dean of Faculty)

The implications of draconian sickness absence policies was also a concern for several managers, highlighting once again the balancing act many appear to be performing between managing productivity and concern for the welfare of staff. One manager described an amount of discretion available to her – a sensible policy on the face of it. However, the experience of this discretion is to make her responsible for managing the disparate interests of the organization on the one hand and her staff on the other:

> ... the line manager does have discretion. So I think, well, that person has had those three days, separate periods of absence, but I can see why that is, it's quite legitimate, then you can waive that monitoring process. So there's some flexibility in that. It's difficult to say what is and what isn't disruptive, I mean the odd day here and there is nuisance value. You know, if I know someone's ... if it's booked time off it's not so bad because you can make plans but if someone consistently just doesn't turn up that's when we get the problems. You know when you can rely on someone turning up [and] they're not there, straight away, you know, we're in trouble and we've got to get agency staff in and we would possibly even have to close the [workplace] because we haven't got the correct ratio of clients to staff. (Health Charity Manager)

Whilst acknowledging the importance of flexibility in the sickness and absence policy this particular manager must always temper this sympathetic approach with the attendant problems for the 'normal' functioning of the workplace. So even though the question she was asked was directly about her organizations policy towards sickness absence she quite quickly moved to explaining that absence can cause significant disruption.

Reactions to levels of disruption varied widely across our interviewees. Whilst some took personal responsibility for covering the work of others' work when they were absent, some managers did not. In an interview with a manager in the voluntary sector, the frustration some managers felt with people who were off sick rose to the surface:

> This person doesn't like what her job has changed into and first of all tried to get her local councillors to interfere in changing the policies of her organization, which she doesn't think we know that's what she did, but I do know that's what she did; and then because she did have a, you know reason for sickness due to mental health and stress about eighteen months ago, has suddenly popped up and said 'well because of all this you've brought back all my stress and metal health problems.' Fuck off. And. You know, I'm faced with a situation where, because I don't know what we're going to do about this, we're going to have to sort it out in the next week or so, but, you know, I'm inclined towards the fact that I'm going to follow every procedure, I will, whatever, and I will prove that she's in no time over the last eighteen months ever raised this issue that . . . that was the agreement she must do in returning to her work interview and I'll go through all that shit, you know because it's about the fact that she just doesn't want to do . . . well tough shit, that's what you get paid for. I'm sorry, you're not paid to just come to work and just have a nice time and do what you want to do, are you? (Community Development Manager)

The suspicion that many people 'swing the lead' or exaggerate complaints to get time off work was expressed in many of the interviews. As has been suggested many managers were anxious about their capacity to recognize or cope with staff that were suffering mental health difficulties and this anxiety was heightened by the suspicion that some staff were not being entirely honest about their problems. As one interviewee put it, 'it used to be back problems but now it's stress' that people use as an excuse to get time off work.

The management of sick leave exposes the tension between wanting the best for the employee and doing the best for the organization, and demonstrated clearly that these two concerns are distinct. This contradicts much of the good management literature which states that the concerns of the employees are the concerns of the organization. Our study suggests that the concerns of employees are often *of* concern to the organization.

Mental Health Literacy

From our perspective middle management in twenty-first century Britain is not a particularly healthy position to be in. That said the stresses and strains faced by this strata of the workforce do not generally have the attendant problem of exceptionally low wages and it would be remiss not to acknowledge this fact.

As we have briefly described, there are numerous tensions that mark the territory by which people manage and are managed – and generally these are not sensitive to the mental health needs of the working population. As we have suggested throughout the book patterns of contemporary work accentuate, exacerbate or create the problems that people experience – and it seems to us that those charged with dealing with people on a day to day basis, the middle managers, are prey to similar problems as those that they manage and are generally ill equipped or supported to deal with their own or others' difficulties. A key concern is levels of comfort or knowledge that people have with managing mental health.

The familiarity or comfort people had with issues of mental health varied across the people that we spoke to. It is also fair to say that there was no uniform pattern where people in one sector appeared more or less knowledgeable than those in a different sector. Whilst a limited number of people displayed a great awareness of issues surrounding mental health many were less certain in their responses to such questions. A manager in Human Resources responded to the question 'what does mental health mean to you'? by saying 'I have to say I've not actually given it a lot of thought'.

It was often the case that those who did not appear to have a great deal of knowledge about issues of mental health conflated it with learning disabilities and then spoke about these two sets of concerns as one. Having explained that she had no specific dealings with people with 'learning difficulties-mental health' one manager said 'I manage the staff but they're just a mixed bag, they don't have specific mental health issues' (Health Mentoring Organization Manager). Whilst it could be the case that this manager does not have staff who are struggling with their mental health, those who did have more experience tended not to make assumptions about the well-being of those that they managed.

Another interviewee highlighted the confusion that knowledge of a condition would cause them:

> If I had two people to choose from and there was nothing between them, but one told me that they had a depressive illness or any kind of mental health problem, I'd be stumped. I would be stumped. (Recruitment Consultancy Manager)

Even those managers experienced in dealing with mental health issues as part of the remit of their job expressed concern about their judgement when it came to their own staff. One example was from the voluntary sector where a manager, after explaining about a worker that she felt was using 'stress' as an 'exit strategy' came to the end of the story and said 'So I don't think people generally believed that it was real mental health problems, and what if it was? What if we got that wrong?' (Children's Charity Manager). The confidence with which the managers spoke about their own feelings of competence to adequately accommodate people who were struggling was generally not high. The appropriateness of courses of action and the capacity to identify problems appeared to cause concern. In a particularly illuminating passage one manager described a situation:

> You know we have one staff person who goes off on one occasionally, just loses it and it's amusing, but if it happened all the time, it would be interesting. I don't know that people would tolerate it. (Children's Charity Manager)

Whilst the interviewee was honestly appraising a situation in their workplace it is clear that responsibility for managing behaviour lies with the individual that is suffering. If, as is implied here, there is a level of behaviour which is tolerated – it can be accommodated. However, there was an indication from this manager that there could be a level of disruption that could not be tolerated but in this circumstance it is up to the individual to find out what that is and moderate their behaviour accordingly. The manager need only manage once behaviours have become intolerable – perhaps too late for a simple and supportive mechanism for continuing work. This again relates to the level of training or competence managers felt they had for dealing with such difficult situations. It also highlights the difficult position of the employee who, whilst struggling with their own issues, must find a way of moderating their behaviour to an estimation of what might be acceptable.

This theme is picked up elsewhere, but the point is that the contexts within which managers manage is one distinguished by a tension between doing the best for people from a position of relative impotence – the needs are not known and the capacity to do anything about an unhealthy environment is limited by the pressures of productivity.

Line Managers, Policy and Practice

In conjunction with the HSE management standards, the 1995 Disability Discrimination Act (DDA) made it unlawful to discriminate against people in connection with employment. Under this Act, mental impairment was considered a disability should it have a long-term adverse effect on the ability to carry out normal day to day activities. This discrimination referred to the offering of employment, terms of employment, opportunities for promotion and training, and crucially, 'dismissing him or subjecting him to any other detriment'. Examples of steps that might be taken in relation to aiding a disabled person in work include allocating some of the disabled person's duties to another person, altering his work hours and allowing him to be absent for rehabilitation, assessment or treatment. It should be noted that this legislation does not apply in relation to an employer that has fewer than 20 employees (Disability Discrimination Act, 1995).

Managers were asked about their own company strategies and policies for addressing the needs of workers with mental health difficulties and about their previous awareness and experience of using HSE management standards and DDA legislation. The following accounts provide a flavour of the general responses to questions of policy and legislation in the workplace.

> I think the difficulty is that, and I probably wouldn't have said this a couple of years ago, and this is where cynicism sort of starts to creep in, but I think the difficulty is that the gap between government saying this is what we should be doing, and actually what you can do on the ground and what people believe and what priorities are, is vast. (Senior executive B in London mental health trust)

> There are lots of umm, there are lots of big policies and umm there are probably lots of well-meaning policies, I just think that actually, when you're on the ground and kind of facing those sorts of things, umm. (University Dean of Faculty)

> Yeah, I mean, you've got the process on one side, but then you've got the sort of common sense approach which is what you'll end up doing, you know! (Department of Work and Pensions Line Manager)

> Whether some of the big companies, and lets just you know say a few, . . . people like JP Morgan, Barclays, Coca Cola, Mars all these . . . they would have the procedures there probably; but there's procedures and there's reality. (Human Resources Consultant in the private sector)

The quotes above appear to provide a distinct demarcation between the information that managers are provided with and the reality of life in the workplace. Policy on mental health was seen to be anathema to the practices and social relations of decision making. Not infrequently policy was presented as somehow out of touch with 'common sense' or 'reality' and that it was this common sense that actually dictated practice. The National Audit Office (2004) suggest that good line managers should support attendance by providing a good communication of policy and health promotion and that there should be in place 'policies and procedures to adequately support employees' (HSE, 2005). However, we found little that resonated with these suggestions. There was also a recommendation that employees are offered flexible working, job sharing and annualized hours in order to enable a better work/life balance. However, the capacity of managers and indeed organizations to provide these kinds of adjustments is not always practical in the currently prevailing neoliberal rationality that dictates workplace norms. Taylor *et al.* (2003) suggests that consciously or unconsciously managers have embraced neoliberalism and its imperatives leading to new workplace norms where work intensification has become a habitual and inescapable necessity. These cultures of productivity, combined with a clear lack of belief in mental health policy, mean that, as a number of managers commented, the 'solution's' to staff mental health problems tended to be idiosyncratic and at the mercy of the capacity to respond. In practice it was often constructed as being 'down to the line manager' rather than to policy objectives, suggestions or legislation. Indeed, one manager noted that 'if it's a good line manager they support the person, get assistance and support. If it's a bad line manager in terms of how they support people, they don't'.

In most workplaces line managers played a key role or were solely responsible for absence management. Although a number of managers subscribed to the school of thought that much policy was impractical or a bore, and a poor relationship to the workplace needs of the staff, it was also clear that a considerable number of managers showed no actual knowledge either of their own organizational policies or government legislation. This is particularly important because the National Audit Office (2004) state that 'good line management is the key to staff feeling valued and involved' and essential for absence management. Moreover, the HSE standards, that rely solely on managerial prerogative (Taylor *et al.*, 2003), suggest that 'managers will now have to work with you to find solutions, so your problems should reduce over time' (HSE, 2005). Therefore, it is a concern that only 25 % of managers were aware of procedures in their organizations for 'dealing with employees with mental health problems' (Shift, 2007). This might partly account for why Sainsbury *et al.* (2008) found that few employees were optimistic about what their line manager was able or prepared to do for them. A majority of our participants had not come across the HSE management standards and a number were unaware of their own organizational policies.

> I don't actually know. We have an employee handbook but it doesn't in any way mention mental health. (Senior Manager in a communications company)

> (On HSE management standards): Is it to do with mental health? (UK University Line Manager)

> HSE Management standards? No! I probably should be! But no! (Senior Executive in London Mental Health Trust)

> I'm aware of the Health and Safety Executive, but not specifically with regard to Management Standards. Again, I've got a HR Manager who advises me on matters like that, I'm confident that she is aware of it! [Laughs]. (Police Chief Constable)

Some participants who were aware of their mental health procedures constructed them as having being co-opted to address the organizations' needs regarding legal protection as opposed to supporting the mental health of employees. As such, counsellors or company doctors were quite clearly positioned as either a disciplinary resource for managers or a self-protection measure even though these same health professionals had at other times during the interview been characterized as providers of key health support for employees.

> No, we have, well we have a company doctor, not employed by us obviously but retained, and they are at our disposal if we feel the need. Although I have to say that in most cases it's actually more for our benefit in terms of potential disciplinaries and second opinions and things like that. It's not so much sort of a resource that people can just tap into when they want. (Chief Executive of an animal charity)

> We have access to a counsellor that we can recommend to people with a particular personal crisis going on; so rather than just occupational health, that's kind of covering our arse to be honest. (Assistant Head Teacher of a secondary school)

While the accounts above suggest a potentially problematic lack of knowledge or disrespect for much of the key legislation and policy that guides the context for mental health in the workplace, there was little evidence overall to suggest that this was due to deliberative processes to render knowable and legitimate certain modes of social practice in organizations. It is just as possible that much of the key policy legislation had yet to effectively cascade to a majority of organizations in the area. However, the suggestion that much of this policy on discrimination, control, flexibility and support, and role consultation was somehow unworkable or poorly aligned with the practices of the modern workplace could have had a genesis in the current cultures of productivity that largely dictate the social practices and potential for progressive action.

One way in which this might be reproduced could be the tension between top down policy legislation and specific pressures on line managers from the managers to whom they are accountable that seek to legitimate regimes of workplace practice that contradict much of this progressive policy. Walkerdine (2002) and Gill (2008) note the effects of economic rationalism on the capacity of subjects to present identities that are unable to self-regulate and display an autonomous ability to adapt to demanding work patterns. Line managers whose inclination is to support employees who experience these difficulties are often made aware of alternative means of addressing the issue. We found evidence of specific practices of senior managers where the intent was to inculcate in line managers modes of action that constituted a direct challenge to progressive policy and legislation. A considerable number of line managers alluded to the pressure for the delivery of productivity targets as a means through which to justify the removal of employees with mental health problems rather than face a lengthy and potentially costly rehabilitation and workplace adjustments. Dick and Hyde (2006) suggest that the conditions to allow line managers to help reduced-hours employees are often not in place due to the foregrounding of short-term operational goals. We would suggest that this extends to helping employees with mental health problems.

> And my big boss just sort of said to me 'well, if they're the wrong people then we'll have to get different people working for us'. So this is the kind of... I mean, brass tacks isn't it really at the end of the day, they don't necessarily want people who are more vulnerable and difficult to manage, so that's kind of settled. (Department of Work and Pensions Line Manager)

I think it's viewed negatively. . . . if I put on an organization hat, I think that the senior management, if I can put it like that, so CEOs and very senior management, see it as having a negative impact and actually wanting to get rid of somebody as a result of that. (Human Resources Consultant in the private sector)

I only say this because currently my colleague, my counterpart in Yorkshire, he does a similar job to me for that area, is sort of being asked to get rid of someone who was taken on by the old employment but using very straight down the line HR technique. (Civil Servant)

I mean to be honest I was glad he left, not necessarily because of his mental health problems but if I'm honest it would be partly because of that because it was an unknown, and I could never depend upon him and I have to say, the people I worked for at the time told me to sack him the minute that I knew he had a mental health problem and you can't do that. (Senior Manager in a communications company)

Yeah, people who actually own the business, because I was running the business, said just you know 'get rid of him'. I said 'you can't do that' and they said 'you can' and I said 'no because actually I'm sure it comes under the Disability Discrimination Act'; and they just looked blank. (Manager in a communications company)

The managers we spoke to were not specifically asked about their relationships with senior managers but a common practice to emerge from the accounts was that of line managers receiving instruction to undertake to remove employees with mental illnesses. The first quote nicely highlights the positioning of 'right people' and 'wrong people'. In constructing employees with mental health conditions in such a way this precludes the possibility that providing a change of environment or adjustments or time off to recover could be beneficial. The malady is the person themselves rather than a temporal response to a given set of circumstances. In so doing it renders the legislation of the Disability Discrimination Act redundant, but it also constitutes a regime that reinforces capital accumulation and productivity through ignoring employees' lawful right to adjustment and recovery time. Miller and Rose (2008) note that governmentalities are both ways of thinking, and tools for intervening, and the quotes above illustrate the way that 'straight down the line HR techniques', that is, the techniques for the conducting of work conduct, can be used to realize regressive mental health practice. In doing so employees with mental health problems are rendered inevitably and corrosively degraded to the extent that they are not suitable for rehabilitation. As Knights and Willmott (1989) suggested, and has been illustrated throughout this book, too little attention has been given to the social psychology of management control. The modes of practice outlined here by senior executives deliver the means with which to cast aside those who fail the neoliberal test of self regulating and autonomous subjectivity and therefore are thought to diminish the potential for capital accumulation.

The contention above is particularly relevant in the context of recent research which emphasizes the importance of senior management in effectively and progressively managing mental health in the workplace. James, Cunningham and Dibben (2006), state that, regarding rehabilitative processes, organization commitment and culture, the attitudes and values of senior management are crucially important. Moreover, the Department of Health initiative 'Action on Stigma' is based on the key foundation that:

> The organization and health values of upper management influence the resources allocated to return to work and ultimately the ability of managers to implement good return to work practices. (Shift, 2006)

As such, supervisors should be supported by senior management in efforts to promote well-being and safety of workers (Shift, 2006). This practice was notable by its absence in a number of the organizations that we encountered. Such findings provide very little substance with which to contest Manning and White's (1995) analysis of a group of personnel directors where half of employers would never or only occasionally employ someone who was currently unwell. The logical conclusion for a number of senior managers is to take advantage of the increases in non-standard employment, or 'flexibility' in recent years and legally dismiss staff with mental health difficulties on the grounds of 'it not working out'.

> ... it generally transpires that their mental health concerns just mean they're not able to do the job very well. So in that respect obviously we work with high volumes, a high turnover, so people come in and out regularly, we've also got recruitment agencies, we have agency staff ... I mean agency staff clearly allow us the opportunity to say 'it's not working out, we're going to call your agency, thank you for your time'. (Call Centre Manager)

Whereas the practices in this section are conscious, deliberative and based on ideological configurations of 'wrong people' that require removal, such explicit and public acts to degrade the rights of employees with mental health problems are not necessary for organizations to manifest regressive top down labour practices. There was also evidence of management structures expressing technologies of governance that presented as 'getting round the system' or simply neglecting support for basic and progressive mental health practices and strategies in the workplace. Specific tactics of power (McKinley and Starkey, 1997) and techniques of governing (Miller and Rose, 2008) can take the form of practices of endorsement and facilitation (Clegg, 1997) and constitute working cultures that can be more or less conducive to good mental health. The organization and health values of upper management not only have direct impact on processes of unambiguous discrimination but also influence the degree to which line managers are able to implement good return to work practices (Black, 2008). Franche *et al.* (2005) noted that it was essential that supervisors have the skills to judge the seriousness of workers' health complaints and to make appropriate adjustments. While the work in this chapter and the last outlines the potential difficulty of carrying out such a role in a matrix of potentially contradictory and adversarial social practices, it is clear that there are ways in which organizations, departments and line managers can facilitate their staff in addressing mental health at work. This might include providing finance for training (since most managers have little or no training in managing people with mental health problems; Hagner and Cooney, 2003), it might include support in discrimination initiatives at work, creating cultures of communication characterized by realistic targets or to reduce the pressure on line managers whose team are affected by mental health leave or accommodation practices. There was little evidence in our interviews with line managers of any sustained or collective will to enact progressive mental health policy at work.

> I know that we were invited once our member of staff had gone off sick, we were invited to pay for counselling for that member of staff from our fund, which we did, but the university didn't pay for that. It had to come from our local funds. (UK University Line Manager)

> Training? No. I can obviously go to specific courses which are paid for, sort of seven or eight hundred quid, but I can't get my director to sign off for me

to go on a training course for something that, from a business point of view doesn't really concern him! (Call Centre Manager)

Basically Joanna – the office manager – put the project on involvement to our directors and they delayed the approval to the point where we missed the boat and we're not now involved in it. Which is a shame. So those kind of things I'd love to be fully involved with, but as far as I can tell in terms of local business, business actually implementing disability discrimination is left up to organizations who are just funded by goodwill to actually organize it and explain what it means. (Call Centre Manager)

Well they perceive that sometimes they're more productive than others and that they might be carrying them in their less productive periods. . . . But there is also a sort of, you know, there's me as their manager at the top kind of whipping them to produce more so I hit my secretary of state targets. (Department of Work and Pensions Line Manager)

. . . and I also think kind of more awareness that the higher you go up really, because I think there's a lot of pressure on my two bosses to deliver and do certain things in many ways. (Department of Work and Pensions Line Manager)

I think there are probably issues in organizations about our ability to understand why it is that people are off sick or struggling to retain and sustain employment. I know that we do have a fairly, I wouldn't say ruthless, it's the wrong word; I think rigorous return to work policy in our organization. . . . That may put an additional pressure on people if they feel that they are being hounded to return to work early particularly if the person who is doing the return to work interviewing is not overly sensitive to mental health difficulties. (Senior Development Manager in public sector)

One participant who was a human resources consultant in the private sector was asked about the way that their manager reacted to their trying to provide support and accommodation to an employee with mental health problems. They responded that managerial reactions suggested that 'it wasn't really, in that culture, seen to be the right thing to do.' The cultures of productivity and intensity that have developed in many workplaces in recent years have explicitly rendered employees with mental health problems 'knowable' in specific ways. In many cases, and across the sectors, this has tended toward 'damaged subjectivities', employees who are no longer able to maintain acceptable work identities and who in many cases require removal, disciplining or demotion. While these representations were not evident in all of our organizations, they were evident in a great many. It was clear that explicit and implicit regulation from senior management made it difficult both for the establishment of sympathetic and supportive cultures of accommodation and for line managers to effectively support employees with mental health problems.

> Because we've got this computerized process which gives us triggers at 28 days.... I think the bottom line will be that if someone has mental health issues, or indeed any health issues, unfortunately to a certain extent they won't be sustained any more, I don't think, in the civil service. (Department of Work and Pensions Line Manager)

Stigma, Resentment and 'Picking Up The Slack'

The line managers that we spoke to talked almost unanimously of their belief that stigma around mental health was prevalent in their organizations and that it could take the form of an amorphous, implicit and unspoken series of practices that were almost always problematic for the organization. Whereas the previous chapter appeared to suggest that these kinds of practices manifested themselves commonly in the identity negotiations and disciplining behaviour of line managers themselves, the line managers we talked to, while admitting the serious and pervasive nature of these discrimination practices, tended to do so in relation to subordinate workers rather than with reference to their own practices. That is to say that the line managers we spoke to did not specifically outline their own behaviours as non-stigmatizing, rather they chose to focus on the way that stigma manifested itself either from the senior managers above them or by the subordinate workers in their teams. It was not uncommon that workers in the team were constructed as the frustrated, helpless and often naive victims of the consequences of mental health problems. They worked in teams where compassion, support and empathy were inhibited by the increased workload that would follow from a member of the team going on sick leave. The following experiences and configurations of mental health relationships and practices perhaps provide some context for Gates' (2000) contention that workers with disabilities tend to perceive their workplaces as moderately responsive at best, and that many feel the their culture is intolerant of disability (Gate, 2000). This appears to be the case regardless of the work setting. For instance we found that line managers who work in public or third sector mental health organizations reported their beliefs that the stigma and discriminatory practices directed at fellow employees was not mitigated by their previous professional experience of mental health.

> ... there's quite a lot I know about stigma from that end, but in a normal working day situation, I do think there is still stigma attached to that, which is one of the reasons I didn't want to tell people the nature of the illness of this member of staff. (UK University Line Manager)

> I guess in general it would be all the kind of misunderstandings around mental health, so issues around violence, issues around sick, issues around people not getting on with people. You know, all that kind of usual stuff. I think locally there's still a prejudice and stigma around people who work in mental health services who have mental health difficulties. (Senior Executive in London Mental Health Trust)

> Oh no! I think what you think is perhaps there's the perception that colleagues will be more sympathetic to their colleagues ... well, no, that's not always the case. ... as I had that assumption before I came in. But, in fact no, there isn't, there. ... But, no, I wouldn't say that they were kind of more sympathetic to members of the team who have identified mental health issues. (Department of Work and Pensions Line Manager)

> ... I don't think there's anyone going 'oh, don't employ him because I think he's a bit dodgy'. It's more a hidden attitude type thing. (Police Support Manager)

> Well it is ruthless frankly. ... The law firms in the City are quite like that and I was thinking of, probably, although I may be talking out of turn, in any of these kind of high flying places where graduates are having to, you know, have worked very hard to win their place where it's very, very competitive, you know investment banks, probably, the Canary Wharf, City kind of environment. I think there is an intolerance. (Human Resources Consultant in the private sector)

A number of narratives were discussed that focused on the way that these employees related to their colleagues who they worked with on a day-to-day basis. Perhaps the most coherent set of representations regarding employees with mental health problems and the way that they were related to in work concerned experiences of resentment that were related to managing workload. Line managers repeatedly spoke of the extra strains that absence through mental ill health placed on colleagues who were frequently expected to take on board the extra workload. They constructed powerful shared feelings of personal resentment and intolerance toward the worker whose absence had placed them in a more stressful, demanding and unpleasant set of work circumstances. It is possible that this set of relational circumstances have a particular precursor in the ways in which constructions of workers, and individuals generally, have changed with the growing promulgation of neoliberal subjectivity in recent decades.

Mental impairment is considered a disability if it has a substantial and long-term adverse effect on the ability to carry out normal day-to-day activities (DDA, 1995). Employers may be obliged to allocate some of the disabled person's duties to another person, transfer them to fill an existing vacancy, reduce their work hours, assign them to a different place of work, and allow them to be absent for rehabilitation, assessment or treatment (DDA, 1995). This is deeply problematic for the modern organization. Firstly, the short-termism and growing focus on efficiency in employment practices have led to a growing reluctance to replace staff on sick leave with temporary replacements from within or outside the organization. Rather more common is the practice of mobilizing the already dominant practices of temporal and numerical flexibility; that is (Hudson, 2002), an increase in staff hours and/or a widening of responsibilities resulting from the ill-health of colleagues. Globalized work practices have placed a premium on maximizing advantage in increasingly competitive and deregulated employment markets and it is plausible that the increased work intensity arising from sick leave absence, in conjunction with the already clearly outlined trend of increased work intensity, have played a role in building resentment toward staff who are on mental health sick leave.

A further problem comes with the different discursive constructions of mental health conditions. Specifically the ways in which rhetorical and culturally ingrained historical practices have rendered mental ill-health knowable as a relatively painless problem of personal weakness and indolence (Walker, 2007). Indeed, the following quotes from the line managers themselves highlight some of these problematic configurations of the ways in which people experience mental ill health. The following accounts suggest different gradations of experience from those 'sitting at home sad' and subject to 'common' mental ill health to those whose problems are 'serious'. However, since the majority of experiences of ill health at work revolve around identities and indeed diagnoses of stress, depression and anxiety, it is still the case that a less serious appreciation of these lived experiences can be anathema to perceptions of legitimacy.

> It's that sort of connection, not realizing that that can be anything from mild depression all the way up something more serious. (UK based International Charity Manager)

> There's the common mental problems and the more serious mental health problems really. (Supported Employment Manager for a Housing Association)

> And of course, the term mental illness, vary in grades of extreme, and, you know, for somebody who, you know, is sitting at home just feeling really sad, again that's a different level isn't it. Pretty extreme to minor. (UK University Line Manager)

Moreover, and to supplement the above notions is the still common belief that stress and mood-based suffering can be accounted for through a process of personal choice. This is inherent in the finding that 36% of the public believe that you 'have to pull yourself together' if you are depressed (Churchill *et al.*, 2000). These constructions of suffering compliment broader neoliberal configurations of subjecthood. The common perception of choice and personal control is increasingly facilitated by a representation of the person as an agent of autonomous choice, the final product in the Thatcherite hegemonic project of creating self-reliant, home-owning citizens. Gill (2008) speaks of neoliberalism as requiring individuals to narrate their life stories as deliberative choices and of the centrality of autonomy and rational entrepreneurship. These representations of the self-regulating subject, in thrall to the multiple choices of consumption, are contradicted by the lived experiences of mental ill-health, characterized as they often are by invisibility, powerlessness and perceptions of illegitimacy. This combination of beliefs about choice, constructions of self-regulating personhood and changing cultures of flexibility and work intensity have an outlet in perceived and enacted resentment.

> So suddenly I suppose human nature is to start looking around and think well who else is affecting my work flow? But that's perhaps, you know, the way of the world even in civil service terms. (Department Of Work and Pensions Line Manager)

I've got quite a lot of experience of that happening and that's when I think resentment builds up and that's when relationships become much more difficult. (Senior Executive B in London Mental Health Trust)

But what's interesting is sometimes when someone's performance starts slacking off and, as a manager, you start giving some of that work that that person's not performing to other people in the team, then things start to get a little bit different. In that bad feelings can arise, you know, 'why am I having to do work for them?' even though they're best buddies'. (Line Manager in communications company)

I've dealt with a sort of ostracizing of somebody because they can't cope, and you know that kind of thing, well we're going to get on with it anyway but actually the group dynamic starts getting angry ... sometimes those managers agree with that kind of ostracism and sometimes they don't. (University Dean of Faculty)

I think amongst the wider community it's harder. I think there is less understanding, I think sometimes there is a lot of resentment. (UK University Line Manager)

(On an employee on sick leave returning to a resentful working environment) I know that ... they will go back into a bloodbath again and have another breakdown. (UK based International Charity Manager)

You know we have one staff person who goes off on one occasionally, just loses it and it's amusing but if it happened all the time, it would be interesting. I don't know that people would tolerate it, well they would tolerate it and that would be the problem. They would rumble underground, they wouldn't come out and say I'm fed up with it, you know, don't take advantage of us like that. They wouldn't say that. (Manager in a Children's Disability Charity)

On return to work this resentment is visited on the employee in question in different ways. As the account above shows, these are not always explicit and public. Where previously the workplace could act as a source of personal satisfaction and an extended social network (Hutchison, 2005), employees returning to work are now frequently subject to comments about the smooth running of the organization in their absence (Stuart, 2004) from colleagues who are frequently managing conflicting representations of affection, friendship and resentment over the consequences of the absence (Franche *et al.*, 2005).When Ylipaavalniemi *et al.* (2005) note that poor team climate is the strongest predictor of depression in workers regardless of age, sex and income one can appreciate the potential effect of these experiences of resentment in environments where line managers often have neither the time nor the training to manage these sources of conflict (Hagner and Cooney, 2003; Sainsbury *et al.*, 2008).

Visibility and Playing the System

Crucial to Foucault's view on normalization is the notion of visibility and there were accounts from our line managers that suggested that visibility was an important element in the ways in which absent colleagues were constructed. In the absence of any outward physical symptoms or distress, and in conjunction with neoliberal conceptions of personhood, autonomy and work flexibility, many employees experience the necessity to perform practices of return to work that make clear an aversion to 'taking advantage of the system' and hence dissuade accusations of illegitimacy (Eakin, 2005). The proliferation of normalizing gazes that establish the parameters of deviance (McKinlay and Starkey, 1997) ensure proper ways in which mental health illness identities should be enacted both inside and outside the organization. Practices of scrutiny and surveillance dictate the appropriate illness behaviour and visibility. However, practices of visibility do not impinge only on those who are 'sick'. The ways in which people are visible or invisible are key to establishing effective, reliable and legitimate work identities that are coherent with the culture of working practices inherent in their organization.

> There are two things that are going on. It's kind of like people need to show how busy they are all the time, and the fact that their boundaries between work and home/leisure are blurred. I don't like that at all. (University Dean of Faculty)

> ... if you're not seen to be coping then people end up getting very suspect and feeling unsafe. Can you rely on them to get you out of a sticky situation and that kind of stuff? (Civil Servant Manager)

> A lot of the stress is not post-traumatic stress, a lot of it is working long hours, a culture of having to be seen, it's more of a management stress that

you get into probably more than any other workplace I would say. (Manager in the Police)

Regarding employees with mental health problems on sick leave, it is clear that they are rarely permitted to be publicly visible lest they be accused of illegitimacy. As a mode of suffering so often lacking visible signifiers, living publicly has come to take on particular significance as a contradiction of what is and should be possible for the employee on sickness absence. Goffman (1959) suggests that together people in a given group contribute to an overall definition of a situation which involves a real agreement as to whose claims concerning which issues will be temporarily honoured. He notes that we are often unaware in our own Anglo-American societies that everyday performances very often have to pass a strict test of aptness, fitness, propriety and decorum, that is, the right 'way to be' for a any given set of circumstances. Mental health, despite its often lack of visible signifiers, is constituted by correct ways to act as an employee in an organization and when an employee on sick leave fails to follow these prescribed behaviours 'we are always ready to pounce on the chinks in his symbolic armour in order to discredit his pretensions' (Goffman, 1959).

> . . . because it's not a visual disability then it does have an impact in terms of giving stresses to the team and how the team functions, and how as a manager you can manage that person because you are opening up these different working practices, different ways of working basically. [Worker with a job recruitment agency specifically for people with a history of mental ill-health] I think he had about 28 days off with stress and depression. And basically, we sort of saw, he lived locally, he was kind of seen in the high street, but you know, he hadn't broken his leg, you know, I'm sure he could go out to Woolworths if he wanted to, you know. But he couldn't sort of manage the sort of machinations of what we were doing. . . . But he was kind of seen and spotted and colleagues didn't like that very much and sort of said, you know, 'well, if he's well enough, you know, I saw him in the pub the other night and he's well enough to be there'. (Department of Work and Pensions Line Manager)

> . . . sometimes in a difficult situation there when, you know, someone appears as right as rain to you; all of their mates and friends and colleagues in the voluntary sector have seen them out clubbing every weekend for the last kind of 2 months, you know they're down the beach, you've seen them down the town centre, they were at the gig that you were at last night and they're still claiming that they're off sick . . . but they've got a doctor's note

saying they're too sick to return to work. (Manager at a community development organization)

I don't think I'll come back to work because I don't think I could do this,' well you know, you've just sat here and explained to me this that and the other quite lucidly and all the rest of it so why can't you? If you can do it here you can do it there can't you. (Voluntary Sector Manager)

The social nature of organizations and the broader cultures from which they draw produce elaborate discourses of information/knowledge and this knowledge can be, and often is, used to constitute acceptable and deviant modes of behaviour. For an experience of suffering without visible symptoms it is people's behavioural practices, visible behaviours of suffering and of recovery that are used to mould an understanding of acceptable practice. In the context of mental health at work, those who fall outside of what are in practice tightly prescribed terms of agreement fall prey to disciplinary social practices embodied not only by line managers (Clegg, 1997) but by colleagues and work friends. It is because of the very lack of outward physical signifiers of illness and in line with Reid *et al.'s* (1991) work on repetitive strain injury, other practices come to take on significance in understanding both the legitimacy and rationale for sick leave, and as moments through which discourse can act to construct particular notions of the truth about a person's illness. The discourses that inform this disciplinary surveillance allow heuristical codes of practice that guide the mental health sufferer into appropriate illness identities and ways in which to live. A primary notion which guides the ways in which to be appropriately ill is that of the all-suffering and house-bound invalid whose inability to perform the duties of work automatically negates the possibility of other non-housebound activity. To transgress this accepted regime for an illness is a contravention of appropriate medical recovery and runs the risk of being identified with the growing number of benefit fraudsters ever prevalent in the UK right wing press.

Therefore, for some employees on sick leave, the price to pay for the increased workload and resentment of colleagues and managers is the loss of their public freedom until such times as they are able to return to the organization and resume their role. These codes of practice, and the associated social retribution and resentment of co-workers enacted on return to work should they reject the 'appropriate' practices of visibility, have the effect of reinforcing a public understanding that a return to the workplace is a necessary precursor of a return to the right to be socially visible.

We also found evidence of a group of employees who were considered to be actively 'playing the system.' In the previous chapter we discussed the way that employees, on return to work following sick leave, frequently experienced a reconstruction of their work identities such that they found themselves in a position of discipline and/or reduced social standing in their organization. In some of the examples below we have a set of contentions regarding the 'true' motivations of employees who had sought sick leave. In these cases it was clear that previous behaviours, conflicts, desires and ambitions are used in conjunction with a failure to properly adhere to acceptable modes of sick leave and illness identity to construct and reconstruct employees' intentions as nefarious, deviant and motivated by factors beyond mental ill-health and inherent to the autonomous self. That might involve 'swinging the lead' or 'negotiating a handout' or a desire to move away with a partner.

> The perception was that she was wanting to leave because she didn't agree with something that had happened in the organization and so at least if she went off with stress, you know she might be able to negotiate a handout and she did get the union involved in the end and did get a pay out. (Manager in a children's disability charity)

> It was an excuse. She didn't want to work with us, she wanted to work with her boyfriend a few miles away. But that was sort of used as an excuse. (Manager at an accommodation-providing charity)

> I think more often because we work in such a caring profession, and people expect the organization to be caring and understanding about their situation, because it is an ongoing part of the work is the relationships. I think people can actually swing the lead a bit . . . and pretend that they're over stressed and they want to have some time off and they expect other people in the organization to support them in that. (Manager at a community development organization)

> (on an employee suspected of having mental health problems) Because this is entirely off the record and everything I can tell you, that in this instance, I have no doubt whatsoever that the person is not telling the truth. (Private Sector Manager)

... this person doesn't want to do what her job has changed into. First of all she tried to get her local councillors to interfere in changing the policies of her organization, which she doesn't think we know about, but we do know that's what she did; and then because she did have a, you know, a reason for sickness due to mental health and stress about 18 months ago, has suddenly popped up and said 'well because of all this you've brought back all my stress and mental health problems.' Fuck off (Laughs) and, you know, I'm faced with the situation now where... because I don't know what we're going to do about this, we're going to have to sort it out in the next week or so. (Manager at a community development organization)

One manager noted that 'there are jokes within the team about 'oh god, I wish I could be one of those people who just does the six month thing' because it happens all over, so there's quite a dismissiveness thing about it'. (Manager in a children's charity)

There was a common cynicism toward 'stress' or 'the six month thing' which would undoubtedly influence the ways in which the employee is able to re-enter the workplace satisfactorily following a return from leave. When a manager reported that people could 'generate some quite negative feelings towards them because they're fucking off lying around on the beach and leaving them to do their work for them' (Voluntary Sector Manager) it can be seen how these practices, beliefs, rebukes, frustration and resentment could constitute itself as a social arrangement of discipline producing a well-knowing subject aware of the way that *they* are expected and allowed to perform mental ill health. Following their own experiences of observing the processes, the consequences and punishments visited on employees who embody sickness identities, other staff become aware of the consequences of sickness absence and aware of the way that their colleagues, managers and the institution as a whole have little space for those who transgress upon the accepted norms and practices.

Where organizations have ingrained notions of the 'six month thing', there are is little need for sightings on the beach or in pubs or in town to illegitimate mental health sickness leave. The absence itself becomes sufficient in many cases for the assumption of charges of cynical malingering and the taking advantage of colleagues. It is useful to refer back to Eakin's (2005) work that draws upon a culturally ingrained discourse of abuse and pervasive, institutionally embedded expectations that participants in the work injury compensation and support system will violate or misuse or abuse its entitlements. This can frequently lead to ill or distressed workers returning before they are ready and/or experiencing a need to perform their personal credibility and integrity. When one manager talked of their desire to root out those who play the sickness leave system because they 'consider (it) to be theft quite frankly', one can see how these discourses of abuse and modes of discipline are in some cases justified by the zealous defence of organizations against potentially criminal acts of fraud. And so a social matrix of factors including the neoliberal configuration of the self, an increasing capital-dominated scramble for productivity and rhetorically configured deviant work identities in the workplace coalesce in such a way as to enforce and enable ways of understanding sickness absence that are potentially pernicious to those struggling with their mental health. Moreover, these practices are resolutely beyond the need for the expert guidance of trained professionals who, through techniques of stress management and cognitive behaviour therapy, re-educate 'patient's' in such a way as to allow them to grow into paragons of self-control.

Conclusions

Throughout our discussions with line managers the tension between an instrumental response to their position and a more personal response was evident. Many struggled with the dual role of deliverers of corporate productive objectives whilst at the same time being the providers of employee support – support often required as a result of the corporate productive objectives. For many line management is characterized by a tension between a duty of care and responsibility for productivity.

Perceptions of work as more intense and stressful are widespread across strata of the workforce making management of mental health important throughout organizations however, for managers this presents particular problems. Many find it difficult to reconcile their own experiences of unhealthy situations with those of colleagues they manage and the façade of autonomous working only serves to accentuate these feelings of a lack of support on the one hand and an instrumental requirement to exact institutional regimes of sickness practice, monitoring and processing on the other. Once again the idea is one of individualized problems that are in fact structurally bound surfaces.

Further, organization values of higher levels of management appear to have a direct influence on processes of discrimination and these values cannot be separated from the logic of productivity and modern capital accumulation. The ways in which these are experienced appear to follow well established lines – stigma, visibility, punitive judgements and resentment – but the context and scale in which these things are felt are increasing in scope and reach.

In the next chapter we discuss a particular example of the discursive and corrosive nature of what we are calling the individualizing effect – work-life balance – and discuss its relationship to our sense of ontological security and mental well-being.

Chapter 6

Work/Life Balance and the Individualized Responsibility of the Neoliberal Worker

A key component of the dichotomy between work as good for people and work making people unwell appears to be related to time poverty (Warren, 2003), intensification of work, labour market (in)stability and anxiety caused through work. As Robert Taylor suggests 'overwork in our society is seen as a primary cause of growing ill health, both physical and mental' (Taylor, 2001: p. 8). For many, changes in the organization of labour, particularly the flexibilization of working-time, has prompted attention towards proportions of time spent both in and outside of work.

Throughout the interviews conducted for this study we asked people specifically about their 'work/life balance'. The answers to these questions will be presented a little later. However, the point here is that everyone that we spoke to had an idea of what the term meant. Further, there was almost universal agreement about the general principle that there needed to be a separation of home life and work life for either to be relatively fulfilling.

In this section we will briefly examine descriptions of what 'work/life balance' means to researchers of work and of mental health, before highlighting some assumptions made on the basis of popular understandings of the term. We then move to presenting data derived from our project and finally discuss a negative individualizing effect of understanding our relationship to work in a 'work' or 'life' binary.

Work and the Mental Health Crisis in Britain, First Edition. C. Walker and B. Fincham.
© 2011 John Wiley & Sons, Ltd. Published 2011 by John Wiley & Sons, Ltd.

Work/Life Balance

The conceptual separation of 'work' and 'leisure', or 'work' and 'life,' as distinct elements of social activity has, over the last twenty years, become established as shorthand for the social and psychological dislocation felt by being at work and not being at work (Bramham, 2006). There is a large literature on the work/life balance (Caproni, 1997; Perrons, 2003; Sturges and Guest, 2004; Warren, 2004), driven, in part, by governmental rhetoric (Directgov, 2007), based on the idea of flexible working (Bramham, 2006: p. 385; Taylor, 2001).

For the most part the question for researchers in this field is the extent to which our well-being is impacted by the dominance of work over other elements in our daily lives. For example Argyle cites several studies where people's employment is demonstrated to be a primary causal factor in a range of maladies. From increased stress and anxiety in repetitive manual labour to 'work intensification' leading to headaches and heart complaints (Argyle, 2001: p. 98) Argyle and others point out detrimental effects of particular working regimes linked to changes in contemporary work (see for example Felsted *et al.*, 2002; Greenhaus *et al.*, 2003; Keeton, 2007; Warren, 2004). The preponderance of writing in this area comes from human resources, business and organizational literature, where authors tend to concentrate on instructing managers how to assist employees with their work lives (see for example Bloom, Kretschmer and Van Reenen, 2009; Clutterbuck, 2003; Department of Trade and Industry, 2004; Lockwood 2003; Weightman, 1999). In a 2005 article in *Business Information Review* Byrne suggests key systems for introducing 'work-life balance in the workplace.' These include: the introduction of flexi-time; staggered hours; time off in lieu; compressed working hours; shift swapping; self rostering; annualized hours; job-sharing; term-time working; working from home; teleworking; breaks from work; flexible benefits (Byrne, 2005: p. 56). The clear message from this literature is that the distinction between the 'work' and 'life' areas of workers' lives are stark and require institutional fixes that, first, accentuate this distinction and second, enable workers to operate healthily in both.

However, there is a growing body of work that asks whether this binary approach to everyday adult life is justified or helpful (Caproni, 2004: p. 213–16; Fincham, 2008; Land and Taylor, 2010; Taylor, 2001). The place of friendships formed at work (Pettinger, 2005), working identities and subcultures (Fincham, 2007, 2008) enjoyment (Fincham, 2007) and, perhaps most importantly, the observation that the work/not work binary has never been as strong as has been suggested (Nichols, 1986; Strangleman, 2007) are all important factors in providing a realistic appraisal of what 'work' means to people. For the purposes of this book the implications of a binary approach are key to understanding individualized[1] responses to unhappiness at work. As we shall illustrate individualized responses, coupled with a sense of responsibility for a failure in achieving a satisfactory work-life balance, can lead to a destructive form of reflexivity. This in turn can establish the conditions for the sorts of personal crises that are commonly ascribed to work related mental ill health.

Emergence of a Discourse

The term work-life balance appeared in the late 1980s, becoming common parlance throughout the 1990s (Caproni, 1997: p. 46). However, the idea that there needed to be attention paid to the distinction between time spent in work and outside of work evolved with the increasing flexibilization of work and, in the UK at least, with the move to service sector work away from manufacturing industry throughout the 1970s and early 1980s. A neat summary of such concerns – and one of the earliest documented uses of the phrase 'work life balance' – was provided by a commentator in the US, Tom Brown, who accentuated the corporate rationale for attending to the well-being of their workforce:

> A model employee is [one] who demonstrates a healthy work-life balance. In every company I know, the workaholic is alive – and sick. But is this the model we should emulate? Do company presidents proudly escort visitors through factories jubilantly exclaiming, 'Yes, all my employees work an average of 20 hours each day!'? If they do, they probably neglect to mention the high turnover, above-average absenteeism, low morale, and jagged productivity levels. (Brown, 1988: p. 13)

Throughout the 1990s the concept of work life balance became part of governmental rhetoric with the promotion of particular sectors of the

---

[1] It should be noted that we are not talking about the sort of 'post-work' individualization of Beck and Castells, more a trend towards viewing ourselves as individuals despite our structural relations.

labour economy and also new ways of working needing to be tempered with the well-being of the worker being an important consideration in the organization of flexible and 24/7 working patterns. By 2000 the government in the UK was contributing to publications such as *Employers for Work Life*. In his foreword to an edition entitled 'Getting the balance right – working life in the UK in 2000' the then Prime Minister Tony Blair wrote:

> We look forward to working with Employers for Work-Life Balance to promote approaches to work that result in more competitive and profitable businesses and a better quality of life for those who work in them. This is an exciting example of partnership between business and Government and a significant move by employers to harness the diversity of our workforce. (Department for Children Schools and Families, 2000)

This level of concern culminated in 2000 with the launch of an initiative for flexible working (Department for Children Schools and Families, 2000).

As Taylor points out, this rapid growth in interest in work life balance developed in a relatively short space of time (Taylor, 2001: p. 6) and was largely critically unchallenged. Taylor's report for the UK Economic and Social Research Council 'The future of work-life balance' (Taylor, 2001) marked the beginning of a sustained critique of the discourse of work life balance which has been largely overwhelmed by discourse of work-life that offers people the opportunity to understand the relationship between themselves and their work.

As we shall illustrate with data from our study, many people appear to have a sense of what work-life balance is but often feel as though a healthy balance is an ideal inaccessible to them. Through these data we will argue that the dichotomy established by work-life rhetoric is unhelpful to people in understanding their relationship to work and home, also that the way in which a discourse of work-life balance is translated by people involves an individualizing effect, where responsibility for dissatisfaction, unhappiness and occasionally illness resides squarely on the shoulders of the employee. We argue that conditions of work are a major contributory factor in such feelings and are consistently ignored as the individualizing effect serves to encourage workers to think of themselves as authors of their own misfortunes rather than their employers. As has been seen in the earlier discussion, this is particularly true when it comes to middle managers.

Understanding Work-Life Balance – Observations from Data

As we have suggested, our view is that defining ourselves in dichotomous terms – work-life – is not helpful, and we were not asking people about work-life balance to either refute their testimony or to establish a 'straw man' argument. The purpose was to explore whether people themselves identified with the dichotomous rhetoric established by the discourse of work-life.

During the interviews that we conducted with workers we directly asked about work-life balance. What the term meant, how they felt they managed a balance and who was responsible for ensuring they had a satisfactory – in their own terms – balance between work and not being at work. While much of our interest lies with asking questions about mental health directly we feel as though there is much hidden or disguised in our experiences or feelings about work that can be exposed by asking about experiences that are discursively bound up in terms outside of a language of mental health. Work-life balance is an example and as such we used it to gauge peoples' sense of themselves as having a healthy or unhealthy relationship with work. The three key areas for us were:

What is understood by the term 'work-life balance'?
What are the implications of individual reflections on work-life?
Who is responsible for managing workers' work-life balance?

What is Understood by the Term?

Almost everybody we spoke to said that the term work-life balance had some meaning for them, with only one person suggesting that it meant very little to him (Wood machinist). The most common response was that it concerned spending appropriate amounts of time away from work:

> I think it means having a healthy home life and social life in with your work life. (Shop Supervisor)

> It's sort of making sure that even though you might work hard that you also leave enough time to do . . . socialize, and do other things that you enjoy. (Shop Worker)

> I understand it to be developing a mechanism in one's life whereby there's a combination of activity, which is meaningful activity, which is work related, whatever that work might be and balancing that with home, family and social and leisure activity. (Senior Health Manager)

> I think it's getting a good mental attitude between work and life – being relaxed in your home life so that you can come to work with a positive attitude. Being able to balance work and family time and friend's time without having to have either one of them intruding on the other. (Clerical Assistant)

The relationship to time spent with family, particularly children was highlighted by several people – interestingly by those without families as much as those with:

> Essentially where you try to have a flexible approach to working hours and the needs that people have in terms of childcare and caring for others. (Animal Welfare Charity Manager)

> You see I'm a single bloke as well. I don't have a family and I think that's perhaps more of an issue when you do have a family. (University Worker)

The suggestion here is that the familial responsibilities demand more attention – and will require people to be careful with their time as opposed to those without families who will be able to give more time to work. The conflation of these issues – that of family and time was at the core of the flexible working initiative launched by the New Labour government in 2000. Whilst family friendly policies are to be welcomed, the debilitating effects of long hours for those without children are subsumed in a discourse concerned with preserving family time. Interestingly one civil servant had noticed a change in the direction of concern in the rhetoric about work life:

> I think what I understand by it is that it's kind of about getting the balance right between the two, which is that, you know, you're not working 75 hours a week and ignoring your family. But similarly you are not putting the needs of your family before work, which is I think a change really. I think when it was banded out to us about ten years ago, it was very much kind of about the other side, you know, that is, don't ignore your family whereas now suddenly it's all come back the other way. (Civil Servant)

As has been illustrated, a dichotomy between 'work' and 'life' was the overwhelming representation from the interviews that we conducted. There were exceptions. The positive benefits of work were highlighted by one manager in higher education:

> I do think there are really healthy things about working, apart from the salary, you know? I think it's the social interaction, the sorts of jokes that you have, and then the structure that you have in your life, and I think that's healthy interaction that's good for you. (Higher Education Academic Manager)

The benefits of work as being something less instrumental than a necessary burden were recognized many years ago – in the social sciences notably by Baldamus in relation to what he termed 'traction' and 'contentment' (Baldamus, 1961: p. 71). However, the discursive struggle between work as fulfilling or debilitating continues. What is at stake is the extent to which experiences of work are mediated by perceptions of it as either good or bad.

What became clear throughout the interviews is that people had a sense of work-life balance as something tangible – it could be calculated and defined as healthy or unhealthy. It was also clear that there was a relatively homogenous view as to what the concept encapsulates. Finally it was obvious that, whilst people did not let it preoccupy them in an overt sense, many reflected on their own sense of achieving a successful balance – or not – based on a discourse that suggests there is success to be attained.

What are the Implications of Individual Reflections on Work-Life?

Having established that all but one of our respondents had a view of work-life balance, and that these views were fairly analogous, we went on to ask people to reflect on how the concept made them feel about their own working lives.

Those that spoke about their own work-life balance or that of colleagues conceded that very few appear to get it right:

> Getting the work life balance right is often a struggle for many people and it's a struggle for people like myself for example. I struggle with that sometimes. (Senior Health Practitioner)

> Not a good week to ask me this... I think it's important because most of the senior managers I work with, I would say, are working to the point where their personal lives must be suffering. (Senior Mental Health Practitioner)

> Right in the middle where most people sit, trying to make a career in their twenties, thirties or forties, that's the hardest time to do actually do it, it's always the time when you need it; when you're trying to start a family normally, that's when you can't do it. (Private Sector Manager)

> I think that people should be free to be individuals, obviously to come to work and try to do what's expected of them to the best that they can, but everyone needs time outside and an opportunity to fulfil themselves and express themselves independently of work. (Voluntary Sector Charity Manager)

> I think when you're working for an organization work-life balance is very difficult to get – to have – because the culture is presenteeism. (Human Resources Consultant)

For several people the phrase 'live to work or work to live' was particularly important. One health professional presented this situation as fundamental to individual feelings towards work and not being at work. As with a previous example she was reflecting on her familial relations. However, her key concern was that the orientation that a person had to prioritizing one aspect over the other – work or life – was largely a matter of structure which masquerades as choice. In her situation she was made to feel as though she was not doing enough to satisfy the demands of work because she was choosing to spend time with her young children. However when she counted the hours she was working they were up to sixty hours a week (Health Care Professional).

There is a question of the overall impact of a sense of failure or futility of attempting to achieve a healthy work-life balance – an unattainable goal – on motivation. The project of balancing work and life is imbued with failure. The logical conclusion to a discourse of work-life balance is that happiness is equated with something unattainable then work will be largely unhappy and unfulfilling – a distraction from those areas of life that would make people feel happy and fulfilled.

The issues highlighted here were replicated in the other interviews. Many felt that their work dominated their lives and some felt that family life was being squeezed by pressures at work. Interestingly, whilst suggesting that their lives were oriented towards work in an unbalanced way the examples our interviewees drew on to illustrate the difficulties of achieving a healthy balance would refer to colleagues rather than themselves. For us this indicates an expectation that work will be detrimental to overall life experiences even if it is not necessarily how it feels – other people are better examples of where work-life issues lead to crisis.

Who Is Responsible?

The question of responsibility is important for us in the context of the overall discussion of mental health and structural inequalities. It is in the apportioning of responsibility that the reflexive response is found. Obviously, if blame for an unhealthy work-life balance is apportioned away from the self, it provokes a different reflexive response than if blame is directed towards the self. What we found was that whilst people were able to identify structural problems that exacerbated unhappiness at work generally they would internalize these problems. So, despite people reporting increased expectations of them at work – or increased intensification – when it came to apportioning responsibility for work life balance the overwhelming response was the individual:

> I think sometimes we don't understand the level of control that we have over our workload. So I think that work-life balance is individual. (University Manager)

In the private sector one respondent echoed this sentiment:

> I suppose it's down to me ultimately because I am self employed and I can say no. Unless I'm right in the middle of something, I can still say no then, but that's going to be a bad thing to do. (Film Graphics Designer)

An Human Resources Consultant talked about feeling torn, but still expressed her conundrum in terms of personal choice:

> The obligations that you feel like you . . . have outside of work means that you're forced to make a choice, you know, which doesn't square with the idea of balance at all, does it? (Human Resources Consultant)

For one university worker individual responsibility was tempered by the feeling that employers should not put people in positions where their work life balance is compromised:

> I think you should be responsible for yourself but then at the same time if you're in a more structured environment than I am; possibly where you're given your deadlines, then it's so important to the person that is managing you or the person above you in the chain, to make sure that they're allowing you to make that balance. (Higher Education Worker)

There was nobody who suggested that problems that they had fitting with the dichotomy established by thinking about work and life separately was entirely the fault of either their managers or the organizations for who they worked. Whilst the quote above goes some way to suggesting that there is a spread of responsibility, this was the furthest any of our participants were prepared to go. What appears to be happening is that workers, whilst identifying structural impediments to a general feeling of well-being were being made to feel that this was largely due to their own inability to manage the balance between work and life.

The Individualizing Effect of Work-Life Balance

The rhetoric of work-life is that there is a balance to be struck between being at work and everything else. There have been attempts by policy makers to facilitate employees requesting certain structural alterations to their working patterns that might assist in achieving a balance between these incommensurate parts of their lives (Department of Children Schools and Families, 2000). From our data it is clear that people feel responsible for managing this balance and that the near impossibility of achieving it provokes feelings of disappointment and accentuates unhappiness with the organization of their working lives. We think that this conforms closely to a neoliberal conception of labour as being mediated by active agents able to control their own working patterns – choosing to behave in the ways that they do because of their sense of place in particular working situations. We would further argue that this is how many people frame their experiences. However, this is a forced reflexivity – subjection masquerading as choice. As has been pointed out, many of the problems faced by people are structural. They relate to contracts of work – either being unreasonable in the first place or routinely ignored by managers and organizations. They are problems of long hours where intense cultures of work being allowed to ferment. These features of work only serve to maximize productivity without benefiting the employee – as has been illustrated by the data. We highlight work-life balance as being a part of a corrosive individualized process because of the way in which it encourages the view that the individual is ultimately responsible for their conditions of work and the subsequent framing of life as dichotomous. For us the premise is predicated on distorted reflections of contemporary labour. The first is that the dichotomy is overstated. It was surprising to us that so many people in our study used the frames of reference encouraged by a 'work-life' view of experiences. However, as Taylor usefully notes:

> It must be highly questionable whether the arbitrary and self-imposed division between work and life assumed in the concept of a 'balance' between them makes much theoretical or even practical sense. The word in context of the workplace looks like a bogus artefact that sounds modern and cool and yet obscures more than it clarifies about the nature of the genuine problem. In reality life and work overlap and interact. Many people gain meaning to their lives through work whether they are being paid to do so or not. The attempt to differentiate work from life in public policy-making threatens to establish a false dichotomy between the two that obfuscates our attitude to the changing world of paid employment. (Taylor, 2001: p. 6)

Taylor's observation alerts us to the possibility that this lack of clarity is encouraged – either tacitly or overtly – to privilege one set of interests, those of capital and production. If thought about sensibly the interconnectedness of identity, culture and relationships means that social life is far too complex to be captured in bland, overarching descriptions – such as work-life, yet it persists. For us this is symptomatic of the problem with the framing of work in late capitalism. The individual is to blame for the failure to attain unrealizable goals. The game is already fixed against workers across sectors and through hierarchies and our experience of work is one that sets a trajectory for unhappiness and un-fulfilment.

Clearly this is not a universal experience but we are suggesting that the conditions are present for those that feel the pressure of work most acutely. The discourse of work-life encourages a view of work as normally problematic to a fulfilling experience of 'life' unless, as we have pointed out elsewhere, a person is mentally unwell.

So why would work-life balance be promoted and exported by employers? The first reason it that it appears reasonable. As was illustrated by the early quote from Brown in 1988, the discourse is constructed around the idea that this is beneficial for both the employee and the employer. The second is that the individualizing effect deflects responsibility for experiences of work away from the employer and onto the employee. A key feature of twenty-first century working is the role of perception. For example it is questionable whether it matters that, as Doogan found, the amount of actual insecurity in the labour market does not reflect people's perceptions of insecurity. Once employees are convinced employers are able to force ever more intense working practices whilst re-iterating the precarious nature of people's employment – as previously noted, a process described as 'manufactured insecurity' by Doogan (Doogan, 2009: p. 194–206).

Work-Life Versus Strong Attachment to Working Identity

As a brief aside it is worth noting what is being replaced by an individualized corrosive reflexivity. The place of identity is central to understanding the complex relationship people have with being and not being at work. The idea of a separation between 'work' and 'life' can be properly assessed only when a worker's identification with their work, and the relationships that are formed within their working environments have been explored. It is certainly true that there is a qualitative literature that illustrates the deep affiliation people *have* had with their work – from East Anglian fishermen (Lummis, 1977) to American locomotive engineers (Gamst, 1980). Indeed, when talking of work in the past, Strangleman points to recent literature dealing with the 'end of work' systematically playing down the relevance of identification with work or the role of agency in a person's experience of work (Strangleman, 2007: p. 97). However, there are plenty of examples of a deep sense of affiliation and identity in many accounts, and in particular recollections, expressed by people when asked about work (Strangleman, 2007: p. 97–8). Perhaps it is the loosening of this sense of attachment alongside the creation of the long hours, flexible, neoliberal worker that fuels the preponderance of feelings of ill health in work. Indeed in our data there are examples where respondents claim that lack of commitment, particularly on the part of managers contributes to their sense of disaffiliation or isolation.

So What?

Throughout this study the tentacles of neoliberal capitalism touch aspects of our lives as workers in various demoralizing ways. It is clear that even in developed economies, such as in the UK, work is an unsatisfactory and unfulfilling experience for many. The economic crisis in 2008 will permeate and resonate for many years to come and the reconfiguration of the public sector in the UK, the increases in unemployment, the attack on wages and conditions cloaked in the language of austerity contribute to a labour market increasingly devoid of consideration of the human cost of late modern capitalism. We have used the idea of the work-life balance to explore how people understand their unhappiness or dissatisfaction at work. It is clear that many take responsibility for the psychological effects of long working hours and feelings of insecurity – and do not apportion blame either to their employers directly or the structural configuration of labour markets more generally.

Chapter 7

Concluding Thoughts: Neoliberalism and the Shrine of Work

Setting the Scene: Neoliberal Britain

Mental health at work is a social experience. It is an experience that is contested, framed, negotiated and made knowable through relations with work colleagues and in the context of broader political and economic rationalities. The preceding chapters suggest a number of clear conclusions that can be drawn from the narratives of people currently at work in the UK. The experiences of the employees and managers that we talked to unambiguously supported Baldamus's (1961) refutation of work as a normally harmonious social arena. In the current labour market, mental health is a serious problem for employers and employees alike.

The impact of neoliberal social and economic activity in the UK over recent years has led to changes in UK employment cultures that have considerably diminished the status of the UK as a labour-friendly country. Neoliberal political rationality, given form by varying technologies of government, or 'techniques, institutions and instruments for the conducting of conduct' (Miller and Rose, 2008: p. 16), and coherently embodied by a succession of political authorities of both the right and left, have enacted changes that have been fundamental to the experience of work in the UK. Through a quite deliberate discursive and material assault upon configurations of subjectivity, collective labour, universities, schools, media, and the judiciary, the conservative government of the 1980s began to execute their monetarist utopia through the development of a pliant labour force of relatively low wages (Harvey, 2005). Through legislation to diminish collective bargaining, a transition in authority from nation bound political

Work and the Mental Health Crisis in Britain, First Edition. C. Walker and B. Fincham.
© 2011 John Wiley & Sons, Ltd. Published 2011 by John Wiley & Sons, Ltd.

actors to transnational actors, and a reconfiguring of the social as economic, the fiscal endeavours of politicians and corporations have been translated into the aspirations of, and demands on, employees.

In recent years the potency of the neoliberal mode of economic management has continued to grow in the UK and abroad despite proving to be relatively economically unproductive. Indeed Harvey (2005) points out that the wide scale international adoption of neoliberal techniques of governing employment have managed growth rates of between 1.1% and 1.4% over the last 30 years compared to 3.5% in the 1960s and 2.4% during the economic difficulties of the 1970s.

In providing an account of the hegemony of neoliberal discourse, Gorz (1999) and Harvey (2005) outline the way in which an array of symbolic and material processes have led to a pronounced swing in the relative strength of capital versus labour. Moreover, these processes have realized the restoration of the worst forms of domination, subjugation and exploitation by making people struggle in order to obtain a diminishing stock of work of increasing intensity, fewer legal protections and lower real wages. The emasculation of trade unions has also been a contributory factor to a clear increase in modes of work that are non-standard and precarious (Wacquant, 2009). A key trend has been the implementation of wide scale and growing practices of flexibility where employees are routinely expected to adhere to new modes of numerical, functional and pay flexibility. This has facilitated a maximally productive labour force at the lowest labour costs (Burchell *et al.*, 2002; Purcell *et al.*, 1999). For employees this meant an increased likelihood of fixed term, temporary, zero hours and part-time employment, 'disguised' self employment, increased staff hours, increased intensity and duration of work, and wider working responsibilities (Hudson, 2002; Lapido and Wilkinson, 2002; McCann, 2008; Sweet and Meiksins, 2008).

Recent practices of global corporate welfare characterized by nation states competing to provide optimally conducive financial, regulatory and labour market conditions have led to significant concern regarding the quality of the jobs that have recently been made available (Lowe, 2005). The relatively low pay temporary employment sector trebled between 1992 and 1998 and temporary agency workers are now found in 28% of workplaces with 25 or more employees (McCann, 2008). These workers are currently paid on average 11% and 6% less hourly in men and women respectively. Furthermore, the 28% of UK adults who currently work part-time (Office for National Statistics, March 2010) are more poorly remunerated for their work than full-time counterparts. Women working part-time are paid 38% less per hour and men working part-time are paid 26% less per hour than their full-time contemporaries (McCann, 2008).

In recent years a contracting UK manufacturing sector, facilitated by the global movement of sites of production to areas of cheaper labour in the Far East, has led to a further downward pressure on wages and persistent low inflation (Bauman, 1998a; Turner, 2008). Consequently, a considerable increase in consumer debt has been the result of persistent low wages, low interest rates and the substantial increase in house prices and rents. Indeed there has been a steady increase in the ratio of average house price to average earnings of 3.14 in 1998 to 5.86 in 2007 (Chamberlin, 2009). In the UK 54% of children living in poverty are from households where at least one adult is in paid work; a statistic that questions the premise of paid work as an effective protection against poverty (Grover, 2007). While the growth of flexible and non-standard employment in the UK in recent years has met the needs of neoliberal authorities predicated on furnishing competitive markets, it has created problems in the clear and growing disjuncture between stability of employment and stability necessary for continued mortgage repayments (Griffiths, 2004; Nettleton and Burrows, 1998).

It is the conjuncture of these economic, political and industrial events that have given form to the advantage accrued by what Gorz (1999) contends to be a historically unprecedented mass of capital. Moreover, there is a growing imbalance between the power of corporate capital and the power of the people who service this capital with their labour. An increasingly pliant and powerless labour force are subject to modes of government and processes of discipline that leave little space for employees struggling with their mental health. A growing lack of collective representation, an increasingly precarious, non-standard and unneeded workforce experiencing increasing personal debt and an escalating difficulty in achieving a practicable minimum income standard has provided organized capital with the potential to produce and organize social relations of work that would not otherwise have been possible. In recent years the hegemony of the neoliberal project has seen a coherent reorganization of a matrix of political, public and private dynamics and ways of knowing and being. People's connections with previous discourses of work and points of organizational identification have been fundamentally reoriented in conjunction with discursive practices that have refashioned and reconfigured ways of understanding the self. This combined assault on public life, organizations and subjectivities has resulted in particular ways of understanding and interpreting the world. Prominent in these has been the individualization of collective suffering and the implementation of unknown and unenforceable health and safety management standards and recommendations to guide workplace organization.

One of the key consequences of this approach has been the implementation of cultures of mental health replete with practices of discipline, control and identity configuration that are increasingly predicated on productivity at the cost of mental well-being.

Industrial Imaginations

One of the reasons for the problematic nature of many of the social practices of employment outlined in this book is that, no matter how much political and industrial labour is mobilized to produce reductionist compositions of labour as a commodity, it is, in fact, much more then that. It is certainly the case that there has been a transformation in public discourse and consciousness regarding the idea of work as something people 'have' rather than something that they 'do'; as a commodity of personal ownership. This reflects what Illich (1973) calls the 'industrialization of man'; a state of industrially formed public consciousness reflecting the prominence of corporate ideologies and discourses. Advanced liberal rationalities are characterized by the access of industry to a radical monopoly with which to shape our expectations, hopes, standards and identities. However, the reality of people's experiences cannot exist only within these discourses and industrial identities.

People enter labour markets as characters who inhabit multiple and sometimes contradictory subjectivities. The self is complex, plastic, variable and inconsistent and it adapts in different ways to different circumstances and social interactions (Cohen, 1994). As social entities people are embedded in networks of cultural and social relations; socialized physical beings with dreams, ambitions, desires, hopes and fears (Harvey, 2005). Work is more than an arena through which enabled and enlightened labour owners trade the commodity of their work in spaces and relations of their making. Strangleman points to recent literature systematically playing down the relevance of identification with work or the role of agency in a person's experience of work (Strangleman, 2007: p. 97). However many people experience a deep sense of affiliation and identity in their accounts of work (Strangleman, 2007) and it is the very nature of these experiences of affiliation and identity that make work such a powerful and variable influence on well-being. Work can be a site of desperation and misery and a site of personal satisfaction and social value. It can be a source of life-affirming friendships or companionship; a place where status is a source of pride to children, or shame to parents. It can be a space where the dominant means of social relations are characterized by anger, envy, confusion, joy, satisfaction, anxiety and distress. Work can be a means through which to maintain social and economic survival; a means through which to service the paying of rent, and the purchase of clothing and the feeding of children. For some people their current work is the singular barrier between subsistence and mounting personal or family debt. Work can be an arena of paralyzing inertia, where the misery of a daily grind is compounded by the desperation of entrapment. It can be dynamic, exciting, dull and monotonous and sometimes all at the same time.

Work is so many things to so many people at so many different times of the day, week, year and life course. Work is far from being a simple arena of commodity exchange and no relational circumstances bring that more into focus than subjective suffering. Under the guidance of the denizens of neoliberal political ideology, the organizational practices of workplaces in the UK are changing. People are now increasingly subject to meaningless, high intensity, precarious, dissocialized and poorly paid work. This does not provide a fertile context for the provision of sympathetic spaces for employees who experience mental health problems.

There is now a disjuncture between the neoliberal worker as a commodity to be maximized, and the multifaceted social beings whose complex inconsistencies, desires, dreams and mental suffering fail to reflect simplistic neoliberal concepts of the autonomous self-regulating self. Nowhere is this more problematic than with employees whose experience of subjective distress directly contradicts industrially circumscribed subjectivities of work. Mental health at work manifests a whole range of social practices, forms of resistance, discrimination, identity work, bargaining and reconfigurations of employee identities as organizations and employees attempt to make sense of this contradiction with the conceptual, political and discursive tools at their disposal. This is a paradox that even industrially formed imaginations, replete with configurations of what it means to be an acceptable person, a good employee and a responsible colleague, fail to effectively resolve. The lived experiences of mental health simply fail to accord with modern industrial and corporate visions of acceptable personhood.

Making the Social Psychological

The very same political rationality that has enabled problematic changes in domestic and international labour markets in recent years has been central to discursive reconstructions of working identities. The individualized neoliberal self, autonomous and self-regulating, capable of and indeed responsible for, solving their own problems has been perpetuated through techniques of healing that reproduce and organize the way that we understand mental health, recovery and personal and collective responsibilities. As outlined in chapter one, there is a plentiful supply of recent political and academic material that outlines the benefits of work for a person's mental health. It is now an accepted cultural maxim that work is good for people. Moreover work has been constituted as being particularly useful for people experiencing mental health problems who are currently not in work (Gallie et al., 2003; Goodwin and Kennedy, 2005; Hutchison, 2005; Waddell and Burton, 2006). The only problem with the hegemony of the 'work is good' discourse is that, for many people with mental health problems, work can be bad. The experiences of the people in this book have highlighted that.

Bauman (1998b) suggests that the creation of the 'work ethic' in the industrially nascent nineteenth century Britain was a clear rhetorical device employed by politicians, entrepreneurs and clergy to overcome the prime obstacle to the new industrial world that they wanted to assemble. A key requirement of the industrialization project was to progress the culturally embedded strategy of organizing work from subsistence productivity to the generation of optimal productive output. From 'what needs to be done' to 'what can be done'. The work ethic, and indeed the capacity to obtain and maintain a work identity, conferred upon employees a moral superiority by virtue of their leading an existence supported by the wages of labour. This idea of work as morally, physically and psychologically paramount has seen a renaissance in recent years through the policy rhetoric developed to address the needs of people with mental ill-health. The prominence of this discourse of 'work as therapy' has attained new levels of industrial and political popularity because it provides a vehicle through which to wed the increasing numbers of mental health sufferers, many of whom are living on incapacity benefit, to a labour market that is becoming increasingly fractious, unhealthy, intense and unresponsive. The idea has enormous discursive utility since it meets two functions of neoliberal rationality. This construction of work facilitates the exchequer (through reduced public spending and increased tax revenues) and through the preservation of a workforce working under increasingly problematic cultures of productivity. Despite an increasing body of work that has suggested that changing modes of UK work are increasingly problematic for citizens both with and without mental health problems, this basic notion has proven remarkably resilient.

Indeed, not only is work configured as beneficial for employees but it has been suggested that it is a psychological need, a fundamental necessity. Schmidt and Hersh (2006: p. 83) note that 'the ideological discourse of modern capitalism has sought to embed work as an individual psychological need' that 'overlooks the nexus which forces workers to sell their labour power.' This dominant discourse on work as a psychological necessity constitutes any problems with mental health at work as beyond the local and global machinations of organized capital. Whether these problems take the form of a failure to undertake the everyday responsibilities of a job, an adverse response to a given productive environment or a failure to move back into the workforce during or after recovery, solutions must by definition be configured as psychological; individualized responses to individual psychological problems.

Imperative in this organization of events are dominant neoliberal constructions of the self. As well as being autonomous, resilient individuals, people as workers need to be professionally responsibilized. They then require access to the freedom to govern themselves in rational ways and to adopt particular relations toward themselves that allow them to improve/recover/perform in a given manner (Burchell, 1996). Nowhere is this better highlighted than with the corrosive individualizing discourse of the work-life balance through which people are encouraged to be ultimately responsible for their conditions of work. In so doing, the complex interconnectedness of identity, culture and relationships are funnelled into a wholly false dichotomy where pernicious organizational regimes are internalized and reimagined as the results of individual choice. Employees, whilst identifying structural impediments to their subjective well-being, are being encouraged to experience oppressive work practices as largely due to their own inability to manage the balance between work and life. The responsibility for dissatisfaction, unhappiness and occasionally illness resides squarely on the shoulders of the employee.

For those who fail, neoliberal technologies of government are mobilized to allow people to know the reasons for this failure and the conduct required to remedy it. In this capacity, a conglomerate of professional experts such as psychologists, occupational health and health workers are available to make knowable the problem as one of an interior nature. Liberal strategies of government are dependent on devices that create individuals who are willing and able to govern themselves (Rose, 1996) and professional experts are made available to those who have failed to embrace this narrative. These professional experts work on people in order to help them to know their problems of work and mental suffering as individual and manageable through self-care. Techniques of 'responsibilization' are central to the neoliberal aspiration of 'governing less'; teaching people to be responsible for their own health, making sufferers responsible for the problems that they face (Terkelsen, 2009). In this way social risks are transformed into problems of self-care (Lemke, 2001).

The Example of CBT

The increasingly impracticable demands of global and national neoliberal labour markets have realized a diminution in the personal and collective resources of UK employees. At the same time however they are experiencing a clear transfer of responsibility for their working wellbeing. Here the paradigm of stress reduction initiatives and, particularly cognitive behavioural therapy (CBT), becomes central as a tool for rational self-management. Moreover, it is a pedagogical technique of social relations where responsibilizing individuals are taught future techniques that they can use to address damaging cognitions and faulty emotional reactions, to continue the process of self-management of problems of work and mental health. CBT is the perfect technique for responsibilizing neoliberal subjectivities where social relations of production are transposed into individual cognitive faults requiring self-management. CBT can bring about that most ubiquitous of discursive chimeras; that of individual empowerment through which employees can be remade into responsible agents.

CBT is an industrial panacea that cures the emergent problems of neoliberal social, political and economic management. It reproduces solutions to problems that industrially determined imaginations and expectations already configure as personal. Personal and professional identities, disciplines and institutions are firmly staked within the present ideology of neoliberal industrial production and these institutions have become adept at mobilizing their discursive might to denature any resistance formulated on the protection of the social as an idea. As an example of Illich's (1973) 'radical monopoly', CBT is in reality little more than an industrial production process but as with all radically monopolizing ideas, it is enormously powerful and widespread. Hence we have the calls from Layard (2005) and others that mental health services should help clients to return 'rapidly' to work without adequate reflection on what kind of work they are returning to. A call for 10 000 extra therapists and 5000 clinical psychologists without any real pause for thought as to why so many more therapists are needed to address the UKs working and non-working population. Hence we have the recent investment in CBT through the Increasing Access to Psychological Therapy (IAPT) programme outlined in chapter 2.

By defining issues of importance or interest, neoliberal discursive practices determine specific ways of knowing the problems of a society at a given time (Lazzarato, 2009). Central to neoliberalism is a move from practices of exchange to practices of competition as the central organizing principle of the market and it is the freedom of the enterprise and the entrepreneur that should regularly be produced, protected and organized. Individual subjects, their attitudes, beliefs and social skills require to be manufactured in order that they can thrive in, rather than obstruct, these cultures of enterprise. CBT can manufacture new social beings that, through their training and responsibilization will be able to solve problems of social relations, problems of identity construction and discipline, problems where executive managers focus on the 'right people.' Training on new ways of thinking and feeling about problems presumably enables employees to resist the practice by senior managers of performance managing employees with mental ill health out of their organization. One must also presume that it allows them to militate against the understandable resentment and anger from colleagues who have picked up their work during sickness absence and to combat institutionally and culturally embedded notions of illegitimacy and malingering that so often befall the employee. This is, one presumes, to be achieved through rational self-management.

In reality, life at work is regularly colonized by new and subtle emergent forms of domination (Deetz, 1997). Complex matrices of actors and bodies administer technologies of performance and governance in order to reconfigure employees and their work problems in such a way that compliments the power/knowledge nexus of modern neoliberal capitalism. What is needed are sufficiently sophisticated ways of understanding the operation of the complicated social apparatuses (Miller and Rose, 2008) that move beyond the mundane and parsed knowledge bases of modern academic disciplines that have made problems of work central to their avenues of inquiry. Work is a key way in which authorities have produced and reproduce truths about the ways in which our lives should be conducted. Layard's analysis is predicated on a naive conception of mental health problems, of people and of the practices of modern neoliberal capitalism.

But CBT Works . . .

Mainstream practitioners of the psychological sciences may respond to these contentions with the not unreasonable retort that CBT works. That research article, upon research article, has shown that it is effective for improving employee's mental health and well-being over the short and medium term, that it helps to improve motivation, and that it makes for more successful work outcomes. Through the discourse of evidence-based medicine (EBM), and a discourse it certainly is, CBT has come to colonize the interventional space to problems of work and mental health. However, there are two problems with the CBT evidence base that require consideration. Firstly, and as a practical aside to those who promote the absolutism of CBT efficacy, the National Institute of Clinical Excellence (NICE) guidance on CBT emphasizes just how considerable the gaps are in the evidence on the efficacy of CBT for problems of mental suffering. The recommendations made by NICE come with considerable qualification and, perhaps most damaging, the effect sizes of the findings are relatively poor (Mazellier and Hall, 2009). That is, the average improvement in mental health enacted by CBT interventions does not appear to be particularly considerable.

Secondly, and in our opinion more significantly, an acceptance of CBT through its elevation via the exalted kingmaker of evidence-based medicine, fails to challenge an underlying ideology that excludes non-scientific ways of knowing and empowering people, institutions and polities (DeVries, 2004). The prevailing emphasis of evidence-based medicine is fundamentally problematic in the area of mental health and social relations because its acolytes in the scientific community frequently fail to appreciate that *all* science fundamentally rests on non-scientific foundations (DeVries, 2004).

The idea of a practice based on science is naive and unsophisticated. Science is based on practice, on ideology, on dominant discourse and on the prevailing political rationalities of a given time. CBT is currently the 'best' because it is the most amenable to the kind of randomized control trial testing so conducive to the manufacture and distribution of evidence-based medicine. It is short-term, focuses on individuals' thoughts and emotions, and is relatively inexpensive to implement. Moreover, the way in which the philosophy and practice of CBT compliments the ideologies of industrial productivity certainly make it more available to a given evidence base than interventions that require political will and/or costly and widely resisted organizational and cultural change.

CBT is considered successful because it fits the model of testing and because the cultural assumptions that underpin it renders it an intervention complimentary to Illich's (1973) 'industrial imaginations'. Problems of productivity require brief, inexpensive solutions in order to inevitably return people to sometimes harrowing conditions of productivity. As we speak, the IAPT programme in the UK, through the training of low-intensity practitioners, is remodelling CBT from a therapeutic process into a psycho-educational intervention. This less expensive and less time consuming form of responsibilization even better compliments a neoliberal ideology where public spending on welfare and health requires minimization. It is unlikely that whatever tool is used to evaluate this remodelling of CBT will find this new variant unsuccessful. If a person is provided with an intervention that repeatedly asks them to change the way that they think and feel and they are then asked after a given period whether they have changed the way they think and feel, then it is quite likely that results will indicate substantive 'improvement.' Randomized controlled trials of CBT, are predicated on individual change. Instruments tailored to measuring individual change following a process where a 'client' is exhorted, educated and persuaded of the merits of personal change will show just that. In so doing CBT acts as the perfect panacea for the modern neoliberal state. Increasingly difficult working environments with greater intensity, insecurity, and with lower wages to prices ratio, where people are marginalized, resented and where their rights to identities of suffering are contested and resisted because they fail to accord with the necessity of productivity cease to become problems if they are thought about and felt about differently. CBT produces pliant sufferers who are taught to find ways to adapt personally to increasingly difficult social and economic realities. The degree to which the scientific evidence base for CBT constitutes convincing evidence will always be subject to the ideological proclivity of a given audience.

Those who propagate the notion that this nebulous and variable thing called work is good generally do so from the perspective that it (sometimes) provides a barrier against poverty through income. Also that it provides a source of social and self value and a resource through which to resist social isolation. However only one of these properties could reasonably considered as a singularly emergent property of modern work. Only income is dependent on a person being in some form of work and even then it is not so much a property of employment activity as a result of employment. On the other hand a sense of personal and social value, and being socially connected, are potential properties of many social activities and systems. The contours of employment enabled by current modes of industrial employment are not the only way in which to access a sense of value and social integration (Gorz, 1999). When advocates of the 'work is good' discourse wax lyrical on the benefits of modern work, they often do so from the assumption that paid employment alone can provide social functions and properties that can be found through no alternative productive activity. As such, it becomes essential that people are able to absorb the therapeutic benefits of working environments.

There can be little doubt that coteries of experts have developed and promulgated in conjunction with the beneficial work discourse. Moreover, in most cases the roles and responsibilities of these often responsibilizing experts are to enable people to maintain the healing properties of being in employment. On the academic and practitioner side there are occupational psychologies, cognitive behavioural psychotherapies, stress reduction experts and occupational health and human resources. There are also a host of government bodies and schemes like the Health and Safety Executive, Pathways to Work, Increasing Access to Psychological Therapies and the Fit for Work Scheme among others. This milieu of expertise and authority has symbiotically grown to assist, exploit, compliment and reproduce discursive configurations of work that make it essential, therapeutic and of social necessity. Symbolic and material labour has been mobilized to enact a modified continuance of Bauman's (1998a) work ethic through the more contemporary and apposite conception of personal therapy, well-being and gratification. It is clear from our work and from the work of others that employment in the UK is moving further away from this discourse and its attendant partisan institutions. Work is becoming increasingly problematic. Changing power differentials between capital and an increasingly fragmented labour force, and a transition from democratically accountable state representatives to multinational global actors are making it increasingly difficult to build a case for the uniformly positive benefits of work.

Resocializing the Psychological

Mental distress is felt, embodied, material and very real. Mental health and mental illness are social productions. If we think of mental health as a symbolically constituted and interpreted production of embodied stressful social experiences such as loss, discrimination, injustice, abuse or subjection to the oppressive expectations of others it is clear that current social modes of productivity will not ameliorate this problem any time soon. A social model of mental health and work locates well-being experiences within an understanding (Tew, 2005) of social relations in which power is a function of macroscopic inequalities related to class, age, sex and race. It also locates well-being experiences as a function of microscopic dynamics of conflict, exclusion or abuse that can take place within intimate contexts. This book has highlighted the way that such microscopic conflicts and exclusions, so closely tied to practices of identity negotiation, can only be understood within the context of changing modes of capital and labour relations.

Changing forms of work organization and practice have become, for a growing number of people, new forms of exploitation and distress. Workers are expected to be both disposable and totally committed to organizations and that commitment includes regulating their own health and well-being. It is not necessarily the case that these changing work environments and social practices lead people to suffering and distress (although they often do), but what we can be certain of is that they increasingly fail to provide a context for this distress to be meaningfully integrated into working patterns and relationships. The social in many concepts of psychology and employment is so rigidly conceptualized as to miss the relational details in and between organizations. People's experiences of organizations are often complex, contradictory and ambivalent. Unsophisticated representations of work, of the social relations of work and practices of individual cognitive interventions are insufficient.

This book has brought to light problematic cultures of mental health that exist in different types of organization in the UK. We have highlighted multiple examples of people being poorly treated, maligned, resented and marginalized by colleagues and line managers during a period of mental distress and on return to work from sick leave. We have provided examples of employees appropriating and negotiating specific identities of sickness in order to secure what they believe to be the necessary occupational conditions to allow them space to recover. We have presented employers undertaking similar negotiations in order to move their sick employees to an identity that conveniences the commercial imperatives of the organization – this may be an earlier return to work than an employee might feel comfortable with or it may be a move toward a brief and efficient dismissal process. We have talked to line managers being directly pressured by their own management to hire the 'right people' and to remove those who are 'inappropriate' for the organization. Or line managers forced to negotiate the increasingly difficult balancing act of providing pastoral care for an employee/friend whilst maintaining the productivity of their department in an organization ever attuned to economic efficiency.

When our participants spoke of feeling personally responsible for effectively managing their work/life balance, there was a clear understanding for many that this balance was essential to mitigate against the potentially problematic nature of their work. The long working hour cultures, increasing intensities of work and perceived or real insecurity are key to these problems of work that require to be offset by individuals through the mobilization of their social and family lives. Should they fail then it is a failure of the organization of their social life, a fact that many of our participants had come to understand. However, the implications of the work/life balance discourse discussed earlier can be seen to jar with the politically sanctioned work-as-therapy discourse that is so central to the practices of a workfare state. How can late modern work be presented to the non-working with recent histories of mental distress as part of their recovery when, for so many of the working, it exists as an entity whose pernicious consequences require to be countered? One might argue that such a contradiction is fallacious. That it is well-balanced work that is the therapeutic nirvana for non-working people with mental health difficulties and that they should actively seek work and then ensure that a balance is sought in order to absorb its ameliorating effects. The problem is that for most people this is simply not possible.

The work/life balance discourse, with its inherent responsibilizing of the individual is increasingly impracticable in the UK. The systematic changes in UK labour markets and the resulting occupational and relational practices make the notion of the individual agent able to dictate the nature of their work/life balance at best wildly optimistic. Harvey (2005) contends that neoliberal theory and practice are hamstrung by numerous internal contradictions. These have arisen by virtue of neoliberalism representing little more than an internationally variable venture through which to achieve the restoration of elite power following a series of economic crises in the 1970s. Just as neoliberal states facilitate the diffusion of influence of financial institutions through deregulation and then break free-market dogma to protect the solvency of these institutions at all cost; just as different agents in any free market are actually subject to gross asymmetries in power and just as undemocratic and unaccountable institutions make key decisions despite the celebration of strong limits on democratic governance, low wage, problematic and inherently stressful work practices are reconstituted as therapeutic.

We would contend that this dilemma of problematic/therapeutic work is another contradiction inherent to any neoliberal workfare state. This contradiction has been essential for the UK's transformation from a welfare to a workfare state where New Labour's 'New deal' was based firmly on a duty to work (Daguerre and Taylor-Gooby, 2010). There has also been a parallel transformation in the relations and identities that characterize those currently not working (McDonald and Marston, 2005). Through the politics of individualization, disciplinary action and the presentation of work as therapy, the desire and necessity of permanent work is unquestioned despite the decreasing quality, remuneration and availability of this work (Gorz, 1999; Mishra, 1990).

Miller and Rose (2008: p. 48) characterize a transition in authority from nation-bound political actors to transnational actors where a 'complex web of relays through which the economic endeavours of politicians and corporations have been translated into the personal capacities and aspirations of subjects.' Through this conceptual prism the UK can no longer be considered to solely give rise to government and this represents a serious threat to potentially addressing problems of mental health through political means. However, problems of mental health and work *are* undoubtedly problems of a political nature and their diminution will require the political will to challenge, resist and reimagine the central tenets of neoliberal capitalism.

Gorz (1999) and Illich (1973) have suggested radical and collective change in the governance of wage labour and in the practices and utilization of the tools of industrial productivity in order that the escalating experiences of meaningless, dissocialized, insecure and traumatic work can be redressed. At the very least the problems of UK employment outlined in this book require collective interventions. Low wages, disguised employment, flexible working patterns, increased work intensity and the insidious practices of marginalization and exploitation outlined in the earlier chapters are a common reality in late modern industrial cultures of productivity. Friedli suggests that priorities for action must include workplace pay and conditions that protect and promote mental health (Friedli, 2009). Following concern that attempts at redistribution of industrial power would trigger cuts in employment, output and relocation; Wilkinson and Lapido (2002) suggest that new forms of regulation must respond to a variety of problems. They suggest the need for competition-limiting cooperation such as price fixing and echo Illich's (1973) desire to scrap equipment where its effects are no more than a means through which to further reduce the potential for meaningful work.

Thus far initiatives to solve the problem of mental health and work have used as their foundation the generic intuition that work is 'good' for people. The movement of people with histories of mental distress into paid employment has been widely constituted as the problem that needs to be solved. This book directly refutes this proposition and suggests that for many people the very organization of their work, the culture of social relations and the prominence of the discourses used to make sense of mental health make it inevitable that work will fail to effectively accommodate, and potentially exacerbate mental suffering. It will only be through the securing of full-time, fair and rewarding work that organizations will become healthy spaces for people suffering mental distress. Any attempts to meaningfully address mental distress in the context of employment must speak to the increasingly problematic ways in which work is organized and produced in the UK.

References

Aldwin, C. (2007) *Stress, coping and development: An integrative perspective.* New York: Guilford Press.
Argyle, M. (2001) *Psychology of happiness.* 2nd edn. Hove: Routledge.
Armstrong, A. and Francis, R. (2008) An ethical climate is a duty of care. *Journal of Business Systems, Governance and Ethics,* 3 (3), 15–20.
Bain, A. (2005) Constructing an artistic identity. *Work, Employment and Society* 19 (1), 25–46.
Baldamus, W. (1961) *Efficiency and effort: An analysis of industrial administration.* London: Tavistock Publications.
Bardosi, E. and Francesconi, M. (2000) *The effect of non-standard employment on mental health in Britain working papers number 2000–37.* Institute for Social and Economic Affairs.
Bartley, M. (1994) Unemployment and ill-health: Understanding the relationships. *Journal of Epidemiology and Community Health,* 48, 333–337.
Bass, B., Valenzi, E., Farrow, D. and Solomon, R. (1975) Management styles associated with organizational, task, personal, and interpersonal contingencies. *Journal of Applied Psychology,* 60 (6), 720–729.
Bauman, Z. (1998a) *Globalization: The human consequences.* Cambridge: Polity Press.
Bauman, Z. (1998b) *Work, consumerism and the new poor.* Buckingham, UK: Open University Press.
Beale, N. and Nethercott, S. (1985) Job-loss and family morbidity: A study of a factory closure. *Journal of the Royal College of General Practitioners* 35, 510–514.
Benfai, R. (1991) *Understanding your management style.* Lexington: Lexington Books.

Work and the Mental Health Crisis in Britain, First Edition. C. Walker and B. Fincham.
© 2011 John Wiley & Sons, Ltd. Published 2011 by John Wiley & Sons, Ltd.

Bjerke, B. (2001) *Business leadership and culture: National management styles in the global economy*. Cheltenham: Edward Elgar.

Black, C. (2008) *Working for a healthier tomorrow*. The Stationary Office.

Bloom, N., Kretschmer, T. and Van Reenen, J. (2009) Work life balance, management practices and productivity. In Freeman, R. and Shaw, K. (2009) *International differences in the business practices and productivity of firms*. Chicago: University of Chicago Press.

Bramham, P. (2006) Hard and disappearing work: Making sense of the leisure project. *Leisure Studies* 25(4), 379–390.

Brouwers, E.P.M., Terluin, B, Tiemens, B.G. and Verhaak, P.F.M. (2006) Patients with minor mental disorders leading to sickness absence: A feasibility study for social workers' participation in a treatment programme. *British Journal of Social Work*, 36, 127–138.

Brown, T. (1988) Model employees. *Industry Week*, 237 (3), Aug. 1st 1988.

Burchell, B., Lapido, D. and Wilkinson, F. (2002) *Job insecurity and work intensification*. London, Routledge.

Burchell, B. (2002) The prevalence and redistribution of job insecurity and work intensification. In Burchell, B., Lapido, D. and Wilkinson, F. *Job insecurity and work intensification*. London: Routledge.

Burchell, G. (1996) Liberal government and techniques of the self. In Barry, A., Osborne, T. and Rose, N. *Foucault and political reason*. London, Routledge.

Burkitt, I. (2008) Subjectivity, self and everyday life in contemporary capitalism. *Subjectivity*, 23, 236–245.

Byrne, U. (2005) Wheel of life: Effective steps for stress management. *Business Information Review*, 22(2), 123–130.

Caproni, P. (1997) Work life balance – You can't get there from here. *Journal of Applied Behavioural Science*, 33 (1), 46–56.

Cameron, J., Walker, C., Hart, A., Sadlo, G., Haslam, I. and The Retain Support Group. (2011) Supporting workers with mental health problems to retain employment: A qualitative study of users' experiences of a UK job retention project. *Work*. Forthcoming.

Castells, M. (2006) The network society: From knowledge to policy. In Castells, M. and Cardoso, G. (2006) *The network society: From knowledge to policy*. Washington Centre for Transatlantic Relations.

Chamberlin, G. (2009) Recent developments in the UK housing market. *Economic and Labour Market Review*, 3(8), 29–38.

Churchill, R., Khaira, M., Gretton, V., Chilvers, C., Dewey, M., Duggan, C. and Lee, A. (2000) Treating depression in general practice: Factors affecting patients' treatment preferences. *British Journal of Gen Practice*, 50, 905–906.

Clark, D.M., Layard, R. and Smithies, R. (2008) *Improving access to psychological therapy: Initial evaluation of the two demonstration sites*. LSE Centre for Economic Performance.

Clegg, S. (1997) Foucault, power and organizations. In McKinlay, A., and Starkey, K. *Foucault, management and organization theory.* Sage Publications Ltd.

Clutterbuck, D. (2003) *Managing WLB: A guide for hr in achieving organisational and individual change.* London, Chartered Institute of Personnel and Development.

Coffey, M., Dugdill, L. (2006) Policies alone are not enough: Workplace health development in the public, private and voluntary sectors. *Critical Public Health*, 16 (3), 233–243.

Cohen, A.P. (1994) *Self-consciousness. An alternative anthropology or identity.* London, Routledge.

Cohen, A. (2008) Is work good for your patients' mental health? Sainsbury Centre for Mental Health. http://www.support4doctors.org/advice.asp?id=304. Accessed 21/02/2011.

Creditaction. (2009) Debt facts and figures – compiled October 2009.

Crewe, C. (1999) Why has modern life become so tiring? *The Times* October 25th 1999.

Cully, M., Woodland, S., O'Reilly, A. and Dix, G. (2000) Workforce composition and employer's labour use. In Cully, M., Woodland, S., O'Reilly, A. and Dix, G. *Britain at work: As depicted by the 1998 workplace employee relations survey.* Oxford: Routledge.

Cunha, RC. (2001) Privatization and outsourcing. In Cooper, C.L. and Burke, R.J. *The new world of work.* Blackwell.

Daguerre, A. and Taylor-Gooby, P. (2010) Neglecting Europe: Explaining the predominance of American ideas in New Labour's welfare policies since 1997. *Journal of European Social Policy*, 14 (1), 25–39.

Deery, S., Iverson, R. and Walsh, J. (2002) Work relationships in telephone call centres: Understanding emotional exhaustion and employee withdrawal. *Journal of Management Studies*, 39(4), 471–495.

Deetz, S. (1997) (Re)constructing the modern organization. In McKinlay, A. and Starkey, K. *Foucault, management and organization theory.* London: Sage Publications Ltd.

Deetz, S. (1992) Disciplinary power in the modern corporation, in Alvesson, M., Willmott, H. (Eds) *Critical management studies.* London: Sage Publications Ltd. pp. 21–45.

De Vente, W., Kamphuis, J.H., Emmelkamp, P.M.G. and Blonk, R.W.B. (2008) Individual and group cognitive-behavioral treatment for work-related stress complaints and sickness absence: A randomized controlled trial. *Journal of Occupational Health Psychology*, 13 (3), 214–231.

Della-Posta, C. and Drummond, P.D. (2006) Cognitive behavioural therapy increases re-employment of job seeking worker's compensation clients. *Journal of Occupational Rehabilitation*, 16 (2), 223–230.

Demos (1995) *Time squeeze.* London: Demos.

Department for Children Schools and Families (2000) Prime Minister Launches Work Life Campaign. DCSF news [WWW] <URL http://www.dcsf.gov.uk/pns/DisplayPN.cgi?pn_id=2000_0099. Accessed 11/10/2010.

Department of Health (2007) *The mental health policy implementation guide: a learning and development toolkit for the whole of the mental health workforce across both health and social care*. TSO. http://www.dh.gov.uk/prod_consum_dh/groups/dh_digitalassets/@dh/@en/documents/digitalasset/dh_073681.pdf. Accessed 23/1/08.

Department of Trade and Industry (2005) *Tackling over-indebtedness*. Department of Work and Pensions, London. http://www.berr.gov.uk/files/file18547.pdf. Accessed 12/8/09.

Department of Trade and Industry. (2004) *Maximising potential through wlb. case studies from the it, electronics and communications industries*. Department of Trade and Industry, London.

Department of Work and Pensions (2006) *A new deal for welfare: Empowering people to work*. TSO.

DeVries, R.G. (2004) The warp of evidence-based medicine: Lessons from Dutch maternity care. *International Journal of Health Services*, 34 (4), 595–623.

Dick, P., and Hyde, R. (2006) Line manager involvement in work-life balance and career development: Can't manage, won't manage? *British Journal of Guidance and Counselling*, 34 (3), 345–364.

Directgov (2007) (UK government Central Office for Information) Flexible working and work/life balance: An introduction. http://www.direct.gov.uk/en/Employment/Employees/WorkingHoursAndTimeOff/DG_10029491. Accessed 07/03/2007.

Disability Discrimination Act (1995) (www.opsi.gov.uk/acts/acts1995/95050).

Doogan, K. (2009) *New capitalism*. Polity Press.

Dorio, J. (2004) Tying it all together – The PASS to success. *Psychiatric Rehabilitation Journal*, 28 (1), 32–39.

Eakin, J.M. (2005) *The discourse of abuse in return-to-work: A hidden epidemic of suffering*. Amityville, NY: Baywood Publishing Co.

Elinson, L., Houck, P., Marcus, S.C. and Pincus, H.A. (2004) Depression and the ability to work. *Psychiatric Services*, 55 (1), 29–34.

Enticott, G. (2003) Lay Immunology, local foods and rural identity: Defending unpasteurised milk in England. *Sociologia Ruralis*, 43 (3), 257–270.

Erickson, M., and Turner, C. (eds) (2010a) *The sociology of wilhelm baldamus: Paradox and inference*. Basingstoke: Ashgate.

Erickson, M. and Turner, C. (2010b) Introduction' in Erickson, M. and Turner, C. (eds) (*2010*) *The sociology of wilhelm baldamus: Paradox and inference*. Basingstoke, Ashgate.

Erickson, M. (2010) Efficiency and Effort Revisited' in Erickson, M. and Turner, C. (eds) (2010) *The sociology of wilhelm baldamus: Paradox and inference*. Basingstoke, Ashgate.

European Foundation for the improvement of living and working conditions (2000) Ten years of working conditions in the European Union. http://www.eurofound.europa.eu/publications/htmlfiles/ef00128.htm. Accessed 23/4/10.

Felsted, A., Gallie, D. and Green, F. (2002) *Work skills in Britain 1986-2001*. London, Department for Education and Skills.

Fincham, B. (2008) Balance is everything: Bicycle messengers, work and leisure. *Sociology*, 42 (4), 619–635.

Fincham, B. (2007) Generally speaking people are in it for the cycling and the beer': Bicycle couriers, subculture and enjoyment'. *Sociological Review*, 55 (2), 190–202.

Franche, R.L., Baril, R., Shaw, W., Nicholas, M. and Loisel, P. (2005) Workplace-based return-to-work interventions: Optimising the role of stakeholders in implementation and research. *Journal of Occupational Rehabilitation*, 15 (4), 525–542.

Friedli, L. (2009) *Mental health, resilience and inequalities*. World Health Organisation.

Friesen, M.N., Yassi, A. and Cooper, J. (2001) Return-to-work the importance of human interactions and organizational structures. *Work*, 17, 11–22.

Gallie, D, Marsh, C. and Vogler, C. (1993) *Social change and the experience of unemployment*. Oxford University Press.

Gamst, F. (1980) *The hoghead: An industrial ethnology of the locomotive engineer*. New York: Holt, Rhinehart and Winston.

Gardner, B., Rose, J., Mason, O., Tyler, P. and Cushway, D. (2005) Cognitive therapy and behavioural coping in the management of work-related stress: An intervention study. *Work and Stress*, 19 (2), 137–152.

Gates, L.B. (2000) Workplace accommodation as a social process. *Journal of Occupational Rehabilitation*, 10 (1), 85–98.

Genschel, P. (2002) Globalisation, tax competition and the welfare state. *Politics and Society*, 30 (2), 245–275.

Gill, R. (2008) Culture and subjectivity in neoliberal and postfeminist times. *Subjectivity*, 25, 432–445.

Gillespie, N., Walsh, M., Winefield, A., Dua, J. and Stough, C. (2001) Occupational stress in universities: Staff perceptions of the causes, consequences and moderators of stress. *Work and Stress*, 15 (1), 53–72.

Goffman, E. (1959) *The presentation of self in everyday life*. USA: Anchor Books.

Goodwin, A.M. and Kennedy, A. (2005) The psychosocial benefits of work for people with severe and enduring mental health problems. *Community, Work and Family*, 8 (1), 23–35.

Gorz, A. (1999) *Reclaiming work: Beyond the wage-based society*. Polity Press.

Gray, J. (1998) *False dawn: The delusions of global capitalism*. London, Granta Books.

Green, F. (2004) Work intensification, discretion and the decline of well-being at work. *Eastern Economic Journal*, 30 (4), 615–625.

Greenhaus, J., Collins, K. and Shaw, J. (2003) The relation of work-family balance and quality of life. *Journal of Vocational Behaviour*, 63 (3), 510–531.

Gregg, P. and Wadsworth, J. (2010) Employment in the 2008–2009 Recession. *Economic and Labour Market Review*, 4 (8), August 2010.

Griffiths, M. (2004) *The consumer debt burden: A perpetual struggle*. News South Wales, BICE Press.

Grint, K. (2005) *The sociology of work*. Cambridge: Polity.

Grover, C. (2007) The Freud report on the future of welfare to work: Some critical reflections. *Critical Social Policy*, 27 (4), 534–545.

Hagner, D. and Cooney, B. (2003) Building employer capacity to support employees with severe disabilities in the workplace. *Work*, 21, 77–82.

Harkness, A.M.B., Long, B.C., Bermbach, N., Patterson, K., Jordan, S. and Kahn, H. (2005) Talking about work stress: Discourse analysis and implications for stress interventions. *Work and Stress*, 19 (2), 121–136.

Harvey, D. (2005) *Neoliberalism*. Oxford University Press.

Healy, D. (2006) Did regulators fail over selective serotonin reuptake inhibitors? *British Medical Journal*, 333, 92–95.

The Health and Safety Executive. (2005) Tackling stress: The management standards approach. www.hse.gov.uk/stress/standards. Accessed 3/5/09.

Helm, T. (2009) Victims of recession to get free therapy. *The Observer* Sunday 8th March 2009: page 1.

HM Government (2009) Fit for work service: Programme of Piloting.

HM Government (2007) PSA Delivery agreement 16: Increase the proportion of socially excluded adults in settled accommodation and employment, education or training. http://www.cabinetoffice.gov.uk/media/cabinetoffice/social_exclusion_task_force/assets/chronic_exclusion/psa_da_16.pdf. Accessed 10/10/09.

HM Government (2005) Health, work and well-being – Caring for our future. http://www.dh.gov.uk/prod_consum_dh/groups/dh_digitalassets/@dh/@en/documents/digitalasset/dh_4121757.pdf. Accessed 22/3/09.

Health and Safety Executive (1995) *Stress at work: A guide for employers*. Health and Safety Executive.

Health and Safety Executive (1974) Health and Safety at Work etc Act 1974. UK Parliament Health and Safety Executive.

Hudson, K. (2007) The new labor market segmentation: Labor market dualism in the new economy'. *Social Science Research*, 36 (1), 286–312

Hudson, M., Ray, K,, Vegeris, S. and Brooks, S. (2009) *People with mental health conditions and pathways to work*. Department for Work and Pensions report.

Hudson, M. (2002) Flexibility and the reorganisation of work. In Burchell, B., Lapido, D., and Wilkinson, F. *Job insecurity and work intensification*. London, Routledge.

Humbert, A.L. and Lewis S. (2008) 'I have no life other than work – Long working hours, blurred boundaries and family life: The case of Irish entrepreneurs' in Burke, R. and Cooper, C. (2008) *The long work hours culture: Causes, consequences and choices*. Bingley, Emerald.

Hutchison, M. (2005) Walking wounded. In Grove, B., Secker, J. and Seebohm, P. *New thinking about mental health employment*. Radcliffe Publishing.

Huxley, P. (2001) Work and mental health. An introduction to the special section. *Journal of Mental Health*, 10 (4), 367–372.

Hyman, J, Scholarios, D. and Baldry, C. (2005) Getting on or getting by? Employee flexibility and coping strategies for home and work. *Work, Employment and Society*, 19 (4), 705–725.

The Institute of Directors (2006) *Wellbeing at work*. Director Publications Ltd.

Illich, I. (1973) *Tools for conviviality*. London, Marion Boyars.

Illich. I. (1978) *Toward a history of needs*. New York, Pantheon.

Irvine, A. (2008) *Managing mental health and employment*. Department of Work and Pensions.

Jackson, N. and Carter, P. (1997) Labour as dressage. In McKinlay, A., and Starkey, K. *Foucault, management and organization theory*. Sage Publications Ltd.

James, P., Cunningham, I. and Dibben, P. (2006) Job retention and return to work of ill and injured workers. *Employee Relations*, 28 (3), 290–303.

Jenkins, S. (2007) *Thatcher and Sons*. Penguin Books.

Jenkins, R. (1993) Mental health at work – Why is it so under researched? *Occupational Medicine* 43, 65–67.

Johns, G. (2010) Presenteeism in the workplace: A review and research agenda. *Journal of Organizational Behavior*, 31 (4) 519–542.

Johnson, A. (2008) Speech by the Rt Hon Alan Johnson MP, Secretary of State for Health, 27 November 2008 at the *New Savoy Partnership Annual Conference: Psychological therapies in the NHW: science, practice and policy*. http://www.dh.gov.uk/en/News/Speeches/DH_091251 Accessed 26/8/9.

Jones, P. (2003) *Introducing Social Theory*. Polity Press.

Jones, T. (1991) UK men top Europe's long-hours league. *The Times* June 10th 1991.

Kalleberg, A. (2009) Precarious work, insecure workers: Employment relations in transition. *American Sociological Review*, 74 (1), 1–22.

Karsten, P. and Moser, K. (2009) Unemployment impairs mental health: Meta-analyses. *Journal of Vocational Behaviour*, 74, 264–282.

Keeton, K. (2002) Predictors of physician career satisfaction, work-life balance, and burnout. *Obstetrics and Gynaecology*, 109 (4), 949–955.

Kirsh, B. (2000) Work, workers and workplaces: A qualitative analysis of narratives of mental health consumers. *Journal of Rehabilitation*, October/November/December, 24–30.

Knights, D. and Willmott, H. (1989) Power and subjectivity at work: From degradation to subjugation in social relations. *Sociology*, 23 (4), 535–558.

Knights, D. and Collinson, D. (1987) Disciplining the shopfloor: A comparison of the disciplinary effects of managerial psychology and financial accounting. *Accounting, Organizations and Society*, 12 (5), 457–477.

Kuhn, T. (2006) A 'demented work ethic' and a 'lifestyle firm': Discourse, identity and workplace time commitments. Organization *Studies*, 27 (9), 1339–1358.

Ladegaard, M. (2011) 'Doing power' at work: Responding to male and female management styles in a global business corporation. *Journal of Pragmatics*, 43, 4–19.

Land, C. and Taylor, S. (2010) Surf's up: Work, life, balance and brand in a new age capitalist organisation. *Sociology*, 44 (3), 395–413.

Lapido, D. and Wilkinson, F. (2002) More pressure, less protection. In Burchell, B., Lapido, D. and Wilkinson, F. *Job insecurity and work intensification*. London, Routledge.

Layard, R. (2005) *Mental health: Britain's biggest social problem?* http://cep.lse.ac.uk/textonly/research/mentalhealth/RL414d.pdf. Accessed 23/5/10.

Lazzarato, M. (2009) Neoliberalism in action. Inequality, insecurity, and the reconstruction of the social. *Theory, Culture and Society*, 26 (6), 109–133.

Lelliott, P. and Tulluch, S. (2008) *Mental health and work*. The Royal College of Psychiatrists. http://www.workingforhealth.gov.uk/documents/mental-health-and-work.pdf. Accessed 10/10/9.

Lemke, T. (2001) The birth of bio-politics. Michel Foucault's lecture at the College France on neo-liberal governmentality. *Economy and Society*, 30 (2), 190–207.

Lockwood, N. (2003) Work/life balance challenges and solutions. *Research Quarterly* 2003 (2), Society for Human Resource Management.

Lowe, R. (2005) *The welfare state in Britain since 1945*. Basingstoke: Palgrave MacMillian.

Lummis, T. (1977) The occupational community of East Anglian Fishermen: An historical dimension through oral evidence. *British Journal of Sociology*, 28 (1), 51–74.

Luxemburg Income Study (LIS) Key figures. http://lisproject.org/keyfigures.htm. Accessed on 1/8/06.

Lysaker, P.H., Davis, L.W., Bryson, G.J. and Bell, M.D. (2009) Effects of cognitive behavioral therapy on work outcomes in vocational rehabilitation for participants with schizophrenia spectrum disorders. *Schizophrenia Research*, 107 (2–3), 186–191.

Macdonald, I., Burke, C. and Stewart, K. (2006) *Systems leadership: Creating positive organisations*. Aldershot, Gower.

Manning, C. and White, PD. (1995) Attitudes of employers to the mentally ill. *Psychiatric Bulletin*, 19, 541–543.

Marzillier, J. and Hall, J. (2009) The challenge of the Layard initiative. *The Psychologist*, 22 (5), 396–408.

Martin, K. and Cullen, J. (2006) Continuities and extensions of ethical climate theory: A meta-analytic review. *Journal of Business Ethics*, 69, 175–194.

Masterkaasa, A. (1996) Unemployment and health: Side effects. *Journal of Community and Applied Social Psychology*, 6, 189–205.

McCann, D. (2008) *Regulating flexible work*. Oxford University Press.

McDonald, C. and Marston, G. (2005) Workfare as welfare: Governing unemployment in the advanced liberal state. *Critical Social Policy*, 25 (3), 374–401.

McGowan, J. (2009) IAPT- more pertinent questions. *The Psychologist*, 22 (6), 467.

McKinlay, A. and Starkey, K. (1997) Managing Foucault: Foucault, management and organization theory. In McKinlay, A. and Starkey, K. *Foucault, management and organization theory*. Sage Publications Ltd.

Meltzer, H., Bebbington, P., Brugha, T., Jenkins, R., McManus S. and Stansfeld S. (2009) Job insecurity, socio-economic circumstances and depression. *Psychological Medicine*, 40 (8), 1401–1407.

Miller, P. and Rose, N. (2008) *Governing the present*. Polity Press.

Millward, L.J., Lutte, A. and Purvis, R.G. (2005) Depression and the perpetuation of an incapacitated identity as an inhibitor of return to work. *Journal of Psychiatric and Mental Health Nursing*, 12, 565–573.

Millward, N., Forth, J. and Bryson, A. (2000) Changes in employment relations, 1980–1998. In Cully, M., Woodland, S., O'Reilly, A. and Dix, G. *Britain at work: As depicted by the 1998 workplace employee relations survey*. Oxford: Routledge.

Moos, R. and Schaefer, J. (1986) Life transitions and crises: A conceptual overview. In Moos, R. (ed) (1986) *Coping with life crises: An integrated approach*. New York: Plenum.

Musich, S., Hook, D., Baaner, S., Spooner, M. and Edington, D.W. (2006) The association of corporate work environment factors, health risks, and medical conditions with presenteeism among Australian employees. *American Journal of Health Promotion*, 21 (2), 127–136.

Navarro, V., Schmitt, J., and Astudillo, J. (2008) Is globalization undermining the welfare state? The evolution of the welfare state in developed capitalist countries during the 1990s. *International Journal of Health Services*, 34 (2), 185–227.

National Audit Office (2004) *Current thinking on managing attendance*. http://www.employment-studies.co.uk/pubs/summary.php?id=nao1204. Accessed 22/4/08.

National Health Service IAPT website (2008a) www.iapt.nhs.uk. Accessed 27/11/08.

National Health Service. (2008b) The IAPT Pathfinders: Achievements and challenges. http://www.bps.org.uk/downloadfile.cfm?file_uuid=685FEF19-1143-DFD0-7EF2-D8A51B66609Aandext=pdf. Accessed 22/4/10.

National Health Service (1999) Mental Health National Service frameworks. http://www.dh.gov.uk/prod_consum_dh/groups/dh_digitalassets/@dh/@en/documents/digitalasset/dh_4077209.pdf. Accessed 11/11/09.

National Institute for Health and Clinical Excellence (2009) New NICE public health guidance aims to improve mental wellbeing within the workplace. Press release 5th November 2009 ref: 2009/063.

Nettleton, S. and Burrows, R. (1998) Individualisation processes and social policy. Insecurity, reflexivity and risk in the restructuring of contemporary British health and housing policies. In Carter, J. *Postmodernity and the fragmentation of welfare*. Routledge.

Nichols, T. (1997) *The sociology of industrial injury*. London, Mansell.

Nichols, T. (1986) *The British worker question: A new look at workers and productivity in manufacturing*. London, Routledge and Kegan Paul.

Niedhammer, I., David, S., Degioanni, S. and 143 occupational physicians. (2006) Association between workplace bullying and depressive symptoms in the French working population. *Journal of Psychosomatic Research*, 61, 251–259.

Nieuwenhuijsen K., Verbeek, J., Boer, A., Blonk, R. and van Dijk, F. (2004) Supervisory behaviour as a predictor of return to work in employees absent from work due to mental health problems. *Occupational and Environmental Medicine*, 61, 817–823.

Nolan, J. (2002) The intensification of everyday life. In Burchell, B., Lapido, D. and Wilkinson, F. *Job insecurity and work intensification*. London, Routledge.

Office of the Deputy Prime Minister (2004) Mental health and social exclusion. http://www.socialinclusion.org.uk/publications/SEU.pdf. Accessed 22/3/10.

Office of National Statistics (2010)UK QuarterlyLabour Force Survey. https://www.esds.ac.uk/findsngsData/IfsTitles.asp. Assessed 14/07/10.

Oxford Economics (2007) Mental health and the UK economy. http://www.oef.com/Free/pdfs/menukec.pdf. Accessed 22/5/10.

Palmer, S. and Gyllensten, K. (2008) How cognitive behavioural, rational emotive behavioural or multimodal coaching could prevent mental health problems, enhance performance and reduce work related stress. *Journal of Rational-Emotive and Cognitive Behavior Therapy*, 26 (1), Mar 2008. Special issue on cognitive-behavioural coaching, 38–52.

Park, K.O., Wilson, M.G. and Lee, M.S. (2004) Effects of social support at work on depression and organizational productivity. *American Journal of Health Behaviour*, 28 (5), 444–455.

Parslow, R.A., Jorm, A.F., Christensen, H., Rodgers, B., Strazdins, L. and D'Souza, R.M. (2004) The associations between work stress and mental health: A comparison of organizationally employed and self-employed workers. *Work and Stress*, 18 (3), 231–244.

Parsons, T. (1951) *The social system*. England: RKP.

Perkins, R., Farmer, P. and Litchfield, P. (2009) Realising ambitions: Better employment support for people with a mental health condition. http://www.dwp.gov.uk/docs/realising-ambitions.pdf. Accessed 20/12/09.

Perrons, D. (2003) The new economy and the work-life balance: Conceptual explorations and case study of new media. *Gender, Work and Organisation* 10 (1), 65–93.

Pettinger, L. (2005) Friends, relations and colleagues: The blurred boundaries of the workplace. In Pettinger, L., Perry, J., Taylor R. and Glucksmann M. (eds) (2005) *A new sociology of work*. Oxford, Blackwell.

Pickering, M. (2001) *Stereotypes: The politics of representation*. Palgrave Macmillan.

Price, L. and Evans, N. (2006) From 'As good as gold' to 'gold diggers': Farming women and the survival of the British farming family. *Sociologica Ruralis*, 46 (4), 280–296.

Proudfoot, J.G., Corr, P.J., Guest, D.E. and Dunn, G. (2009) Cognitive-behavioural training to change attributional style improves employee well-being, job satisfaction, productivity, and turnover. *Personality and Individual Differences*, 46 (2), 147–153.

Purcell, K., Hogarth, T. and Simm, C. (1999) *Whose flexibility? The costs and benefits of 'non-standard' working arrangements and contractual relations*. York, Joseph Rowntree Foundation.

Raisborough, J. (2006) Getting onboard: Women, access and serious leisure. *Sociological Review*, 54 (2), 242–262.

Rees, D.W. (1996) *The skills of management: Fourth edition*. London, International Thomson Business Press.

Reid, J., Ewan, C., and Lowy, E. (1991) Pilgrimage of pain: The illness experiences of women with repetition strain injury and the search for credibility. *Soc Sci Med.*, 32 (5), 601–612.

Rife, J.C. (2001) Mental health benefits of part-time employment: A case study. *Clinical Gerontologist: The Journal of Aging and Mental Health*, 24(3–4), 186–188.

Rinaldi, M. and Perkins, R. (2005) Early intervention: A hand up the slippery slope. In Grove, B., Secker, J. and Seebohm, P. *New thinking about mental health employment*. Radcliffe Publishing.

Robinson, A.M. and Smallman, C. (2006) The contemporary British workplace: A safer and healthier place? *Work, Employment and Society*, 20(1), 87–107.

Rose, N. (1996) Governing 'advanced' liberal democracies. In Barry, A., Osborne, T. and Rose, N. *Foucault and political reason*. Routledge.

Ruwaard, J., Lange, A., Bouwman, M., Broeksteeg, J. and Schrieken, B. (2007) E-mailed standardized cognitive behavioural treatment of work-related stress: A randomized controlled trial. *Cognitive Behaviour Therapy*, 36 (3), 179–192.

Sainsbury, R., Irvine, A., Aston, J., Wilson, S., Williams, C. and Sinclair, A. (2008) *Mental health and employment*. Department for Work and Pensions.

The Sainsbury Centre for Mental Health (2003) *Briefing 22: Money for mental health: A review of public spending on mental health care*.

Schmidt, J.D., and Hersh, J. (2006) Neoliberal globalisation: Workfare without welfare. *Globalizations*, 3(1), 69–89.

Schneider, J., Heyman, A. and Turton, N. (2002) *Occupational outcomes: From evidence to implementation*. University of Durham.

Secker, J., Grove, B. and Membrey, H. (2005) Recovering a life: An in-depth look at employment support in the UK. In Grove, B., Secker, J. and Seebohm, P. *New thinking about mental health employment*. Radcliffe Publishing.

The Secretaries of State for the Department of Work and Pensions and the Department of Health (2009a) Working our way to better mental health: A framework for action. http://www.workingforhealth.gov.uk/documents/Working-our-way-to-better-mental-health-tagged.pdf. Accessed 20/12/09.

The Secretaries of State for the Department of Work and Pensions and the Department of Health (2009b) Working our way to better mental health: A framework for action (companion guide). http://www.workingforhealth.gov.uk/documents/companion-guide.pdf. Accessed 20/12/09.

Secretary of State for Department of Work and Pensions (2008) *Improving health and work: Changing lives*.

The Secretary of State for Work and Pensions (2002) Pathways to work: Helping people into employment. http://www.feantsa.org/files/Health%20and%20Social%20Protection/Brussels%20September%202005/pathways.pdf. Accessed 4/12/09.

Seebohm, P. and Secker, J. (2005) What do service users want? In Grove, B., Secker, J. and Seebohm, P. (2005) *New thinking about mental health employment*. Radcliffe Publishing.

Seebohm, P. (2005) Putting the community back into community care. In Grove, B., Secker, J. and Seebohm, P. (2005) *New thinking about mental health employment*. Radcliffe Publishing.

Sengin, K. (2003) Work related attributes of RN job satisfaction in acute care hospitals. *The Journal of Nursing Administration*, 33 (6) 317–320.

Seymour, L. and Grove, B. (2005) *Workplace interventions for people with common mental health problems: Evidence review and recommendations*. British Occupational Health Research Foundation.

Shift (2008) Line managers' resource: A practical guide to managing and supporting people with mental health problems in the workplace. http://www.mindfulemployer.net/Shift%20Line%20Managers%20Resource.pdf. Accessed 23/4/10.

Shift (2006) Action on stigma: Employers' views on promoting mental health and ending discrimination at work. http://shift.org.uk/work/employment/feedbackreport/index.html. Accessed 23/4/10.

Smith, H.J. (2003) The shareholders vs. stakeholders debate. *MIT Sloan Management Review*, Summer, 85–90.

Stefan, S. (2002) Hollow promises: Employment discrimination against people with mental disabilities. *American Psychological Association*.

Stiglitz, J. (2002) *Globalization and its discontents*. Penguin.

Strangleman, T. (2007) The nostalgia for permanence at work? The end of work and its commentators. *Sociological Review*, 55 (1), 81–103.

Strauss, J.S. and Davidson, L. (1996) Mental disorders, work and choice. In Bonnie, R.J. and Monahan, J. *Mental disorder, work disability, and the law*. University of Chicago Press.

Stuart, H. (2004) Stigma and work. *Mental Health in the Workplace*, 5 (2), 100–111.

Sturges, J. and Guest, D. (2004) Working to live or living to work? Work/life balance in the early career. *Human Resource Management Journal*, 14 (4), 5–20.

Sveinsdottir, H., Biering, P. and Ramel, A. (2006) Occupational stress, job satisfaction, and working environment among Icelandic nurses: A cross sectional questionnaire survey. *International Journal of Nursing Studies*, 43, 875–889.

Sweet, S. and Meiksins, P. (2008) *Changing contours of work: Jobs and opportunities in the new economy*. Pine Forge Press.

Tarquinio, C. (2008) Work is good for you! Psychological approaches to the problematic of occupational health. *European Review of Applied Psychology/Revue Européenne de Psychologie Appliquée*, 58 (4), 199–200.

Taylor, P., Baldry, C., Bain, P. and Ellis, V. (2003) A unique working environment: Health, sickness, and absence management in UK call centres. *Work, Employment and Society*, 17 (3), 435–458.

Taylor, R. (2001) *The future of work-life balance*. Swindon: ESRC.

Taylor, R. (2000) *Britain's world of work- myths and realities*. ESRC Seminar Series.

ter Doest, L., Maes, S., Gebhardt, W. and Koelewijn, H. (2006) Personal goal facilitation through work: Implications for employee satisfaction and well-being. *Applied Psychology*, 55 (2), 192–219.

Terkelsen, T.B. (2009) Transforming subjectivities in psychiatric care. *Subjectivity*, 27, 195–216.

Tew, J. (2005) Core themes of social perspectives. In Tew, J. (ed.) *Social perspectives in mental health*. Jessica Kingsley Publishers.

Third Sector European Network (2006) *The price of exclusion. European Social Fund: a potential response for those furthest from the labour market*.

Thomas, K., Secker, J. and Grove, B. (2005) Qualitative evaluation of a job retention pilot for people with mental health problems. *British Journal of General Practice*, 7, 546–547.

Thomas, T. and Secker, J. (2005) Getting off the slippery slope: What do we know about what works. In Grove, B., Secker, J. and Seebohm, P. (2005) *New thinking about mental health employment*. Radcliffe Publishing.

Thornicroft, G. (2006) *Shunned: Discrimination against people with mental illness*. Oxford University Press.

Turner, G. (2008) *The credit crunch*. Pluto Press, London.

UNICEF (2007a) An overview of child well-being in rich countries: A comprehensive assessment of the lives and well-being of children and adolescents in the economically advanced nations. The United Nations Children's Fund. http://unicef-icdc.org/publications/pdf/rc7_eng.pdf. Accessed 1/10/08.

UNICEF (2007b) *An overview of child well-being in rich countries*. Report Card 7.

Vaillant, G.E. and Vaillant, C.O. (1982) Natural history of male psychological health: X. Work as a predictor of positive mental health. *Annual Progress in Child Psychiatry and Child Development*, 602–619.

Van der Klink, J.J.L., Blonk, R.W.B., Schene, A.H. and van Dijk, F.J.H. (2001) The benefits of interventions for work-related stress. *American Journal of Public Health*, 91, 270–276.

Wacquant, L. (2009) *Punishing the poor. The neoliberal government of social insecurity*. Duke University Press.

Waddell, G., and Burton, A.K. (2006) *Is work good for your health and wellbeing?* Norwich: The Stationery Office.

Wainwright, D. and Calnan, M. (2002) *Work stress*. Open University Press.

Walker, C. (2009) IAPT, Globalisation and the Credit Crunch: Is this how we put politics into depression? *The Journal of Critical Psychology, Counselling and Psychotherapy*, 9 (2), 66–74.

Walker, C. (2007) *Depression and globalization*. New York, Springer.

Walkerdine, V. (2002) Introduction. In Walkerdine, V. (ed) *Challenging subjects: Critical psychology for a new millennium*. Basingstoke, Palgrave.

Wallop, H. (2009) Britons 'have worst quality of life in Europe. *Daily Telegraph*. October 12th 2009 (News Section) 12.

Wang, J., Lesage, A., Schmitz, N. and Drapeau, A. (2008) The relationship between work stress and mental disorders in men and women: Findings from a population based study. *Journal of Epidemiology and Community Health*, 62, 42–47.

Warren, T. (2003) Class and gender based working time? Time poverty and the division of domestic labour. *Sociology*, 37 (4,) 733–752.

Warren, T. (2004) Working part-time: Achieving a successful 'work-life' balance? *British Journal of Sociology*, 55 (1), 91–121.

Weightman, J. (1999) *Managing people*. London, CIPD.

White, J. (2008) Stepping up primary care. *The Psychologist*, 21 (10), 844–847.
Wichert, I. (2002) The effects of health and well-being. In Burchell, B., Lapido, D. and Wilkinson, F. *Job insecurity and work intensification*. London, Routledge.
Wilkinson, F. and Lapido, D. (2002) What can governments do? In Burchell, B., Lapido, D. and Wilkinson, F. *Job insecurity and work intensification*. London, Routledge.
Williams, H. (2006) *Britain's power elites. The rebirth of a ruling class*. London, Constable.
Ylipaavalniemi, J., Kivimaki, M., Elovainio, M., Virtanen, M., Keltikangas-Jarvinen, L. and Vahtera, J. (2005) Psychosocial work characteristics and incidence of newly diagnosed depression: A prospective cohort study of three different models. *Social Science and Medicine*, 61, 111–122.
Zabkiewicz, D. and Schmidt, L.A. (2009) The mental health benefits of work: Do they apply to welfare mothers with a drinking problem? *The Journal of Behavioral Health Services and Research*, 36 (1), 96–110.

Index

absenteeism 5, 13, 53, 135
　see also sickness absence (sick leave)
abuse 68, 86, 87–8, 97, 130–1, 159
Action on Stigma 118
adjustments 72–5, 90, 142
　policy and practice 113–14, 116, 117, 119
antidepressants 3–4
anxiety 3, 6, 24, 45, 49–54, 77, 151
　duty of care 105
　interventions 18, 19
　sickness absence 110
　stigma and resentment 124
　work/life balance 133, 134
　working hours 47, 50
assertiveness 18
attitudes 1, 16, 17, 22, 31–5, 155
autonomy 43–4, 47, 49, 60, 107–8, 131
　neoliberalism 68, 151, 152, 153
　policy and practice 116, 118
　stigma and resentment 124
　visibility 126, 129
　working culture 63–4, 65–6

Baldamus, W 40–2, 43, 44–5, 93, 139, 147
　fatigue 49–50, 51
　goal orientation 60, 62
　working culture 63, 64, 66

Bauman, Z 27, 149, 152, 158
benevolence 98
bibliotherapy 19
bipolar disorder 71
Black, Dame Carol 1, 21–4
Blair, Tony 35, 136
breathing exercises 16, 33
bullying 16, 20, 100

call centres 21, 29, 50
censure 85
children 12, 138, 140, 149, 151
class 8, 12, 43, 63
Clubhouse model 17
cognitive behavioural therapy (CBT) 17–19, 20, 24, 34, 37, 154–9
　visibility 131
collective bargaining and representation 147, 149
company doctors 115
complimentary perspectives 7–8
confidence 11, 18, 31, 91–2
conviviality 42
counsellors and counselling 18, 115
creativity 48–9
Criminal Records Bureau (CRB) 104

Work and the Mental Health Crisis in Britain, First Edition. C. Walker and B. Fincham.
© 2011 John Wiley & Sons, Ltd. Published 2011 by John Wiley & Sons, Ltd.

culture of work 2, 3–4, 10, 13, 23–4, 34–6, 99
  adjustments 74
  anxiety and stress 51, 53, 65
  CBT 155, 157
  changing 8, 28–9, 30, 32
  identities 69, 70, 94–5
  identity discipline 85–6, 88
  neoliberalism 66, 147, 150, 152–3, 159, 160, 162
  policy and practice 114, 116, 118, 119, 120–1
  productivity obligation 105
  stigma and resentment 121, 123, 124
  substandard employees 92
  visibility 126, 128, 130
  work experiences 39–40, 43, 44–5, 62–6
  work/life balance 140, 143
  working hours 46, 62–3, 65
  working relationships 55–7

depression 3, 6, 12, 24, 35
  anxiety and stress 50, 53
  duty of care 103
  identities 71, 76–7
  interventions 15, 19
  knowledge of managers 111
  refused executive role 32
  stigma and resentment 124, 126
  substandard employees 90, 91
  visibility 127
  working relationships 55
Disability Discrimination Act (1995) 73, 75, 92, 112–13, 117
discipline 9, 79–84, 89, 93, 95, 98
  CBT 155
  colleague reinforcement 84
  neoliberalism 150
  policy and practice 115, 121
  stigma and resentment 121
  visibility 128–9, 130–1
disclosure 4, 99, 108–9

discrimination 7, 21, 31–3, 37, 97–9, 131
  identities 68, 70, 72, 76, 95
  neoliberalism 151, 159
  policy 99, 100
  policy and practice 112, 116, 119, 120
  stigma and resentment 121–2
dismissal 31–2, 90–2, 99, 160
  policy and practice 113, 116–17, 118, 121
domination 69
duty of care 101, 102–5, 131

e-mails 48, 105
emotional exhaustion 34
empathy 98, 99, 121
employment advisors 15
employment records 83
ethics 61–2, 102
European Foundation for the Improvement of Living and Working Conditions 28
evidence-based medicine (EBM) 156–7
exercise 16, 33

Factories Act (1802) 5
fatigue 45, 49–50, 51
Fit for Work Scheme 22, 24, 158
fixed-term employment 27–8, 148
flexibilization 2, 68, 133–6, 138, 144
flexible working 7, 8–10, 28–9, 98
  goal orientation 59, 60
  neoliberalism 148, 149, 162
  policy and practice 114, 116, 118
  sickness absence policy 109
  stigma and resentment 123, 124
  technology 48
  visibility 126
  working culture 65–6
Foucault, M 69, 79, 94, 126
free lance working 47, 52, 59

gender 28–9, 148–9
general practitioners (GPs) 3–4, 6, 18, 71, 80

globalization 26
goal orientation 45, 58–62, 63–4
Gorz, A 26–7, 32, 40, 43–5, 64, 67, 93–4
  goal orientation 59, 60
  management 102, 106–7
  neoliberalism 148, 149, 158, 161
  Reclaiming Work 8, 43
  subjection 8, 43, 59, 64, 67, 102
  technology 49
  working hours 46–7
  working relationships 56

harassment 99
Harvey, D 147, 148, 150, 161
health benefits of work 2, 11–12, 14
health promotion 10
health and safety 20, 150
Health and Safety at Work Act (1974) 5
Health and Safety Executive (HSE) 5, 20–1, 23–4, 36–7, 100
  CBT 158
  policy and practice 112–13, 115
holistic approach 16–17

identities 67–9, 74–5, 88–92, 93–5, 97–8
  CBT 155, 157
  neoliberalism 150–3
  reinforcing discipline 84–8, 93
identity negotiation 79–84, 85, 93–5, 97, 159
  stigma and resentment 121, 124
identity, sickness 75–9, 80–4, 93–5, 160
  discipline 85–8
  negotiation 79–84, 85, 94, 97
  substandard employees 88–92
  visibility 126, 128, 129–31
identity, unemployable 12
identity, working 30–1, 134, 144–5
Illich, Ivan 40, 42–3, 44–5, 60, 64
  CBT 155, 157
  neoliberalism 161–2
incapacity benefit 1, 13–14, 15–16, 18–19, 22, 153

Increasing Access to Psychological Therapy (IAPT) 19, 20, 22, 24, 36
  neoliberalism 155, 157, 158
individualism 7, 40, 44, 56, 63
industrial relations 93
inequality 70
isolation 67, 72, 107, 158

job insecurity 2–3, 8–9, 28–9, 33, 39, 66, 68
  anxiety and stress 51
  line managers 101
  work/life balance 144, 145
  working hours 47
Job Insecurity and Work Intensification Study (JIWIS) 28–9
job sharing 114, 134

language 42–3
Layard, Richard 1, 19, 155, 156
lean production 43
learning disabilities 111
legislation 5, 112–17
  disability 73, 75, 92, 112–13, 117

macro analysis of work 8–9, 41, 45, 51, 159
managers 1, 28, 31–7, 97–8, 100–1, 106–8, 131–2
  adjustments 72–5, 90
  anxiety and stress 50–1, 53, 108, 110, 112
  Black Report 22–4
  CBT 155
  discipline 9, 85–8
  duty of care 102–5
  goal orientation 59, 60–2
  healthy workplace 20–1
  identities 70, 76–8, 79–84, 85–8, 94
  mental health literacy 110–12
  neoliberalism 97, 98, 147, 160
  policy 99–100
  policy and practice 112–21
  productivity obligations 105–6

managers (cont'd)
  stigma and resentment 121–6
  substandard employees 88–92
  technology 48
  training 23, 119–20, 155
  visibility 126–31
  work/life balance 134, 136, 140, 142, 143, 145
  working culture 64
  working hours 47
  working relationships 55–8
manufacturing 9, 11, 135, 149
marginalization 21, 36, 37, 97, 99, 157
  neoliberalism 160, 162
micro analysis of work 8–9, 41, 45, 51, 66, 159
mobile phones 48

National Institute for Health and Clinical Excellence (NICE) 3, 19, 22, 36, 156
neoliberalism 24, 31, 68, 70, 93–5, 147–62
  changing employment landscape 26
  goal orientation 59, 60
  managers 97, 98, 147, 160
  policy and practice 114, 118
  work/life balance 133–45
  stigma and resentment 123, 124
  visibility 126, 131
  working culture 66, 147, 150, 152–3, 159, 160, 162
New Deal for Welfare 15
normalization 9, 126

occupational health 83, 91, 105, 115, 154, 158
  working culture 65
  working relationships 57–8

panic attacks 85, 89
part-time employment 148–9
Pathways to Work 16, 36, 158

pay 83–4, 110, 157, 158
  neoliberalism 147, 148–9, 151–2, 161–2
  see also sick pay
perception of others 54–8
post-Taylorism 43, 64
poverty 25–6, 149
power 7, 30–1, 40, 98, 119
  identities 69–70, 74, 82, 93, 94
  neoliberalism 149, 156, 158, 161, 162
  trade unions 27
precarious employment 2–3
presenteeism 34, 47, 140
primary care trusts 19, 24, 71
private sector 2, 10, 44, 98, 122, 140
  duty of care 103
  goal orientation 59
  working hours 46–7
productivity 7–8, 9, 13, 15, 30–2, 40
  adjustments 74
  CBT 157
  duty of care 103, 104
  identities 95, 76
  interventions 18
  managers 98, 101, 131
  neoliberalism 68, 150, 152–3, 159–62
  obligations 101, 105–6
  policy and practice 112, 114, 116, 117, 120
  sickness absence 108–9
  stress 51
  substandard employees 92
  work/life balance 135, 143
  working culture 63
psychosocial functions of work 11
psychosis 71
public sector 2, 10, 21, 44, 98
  anxiety and stress 52, 53
  goal orientation 59–62
  reconfiguration 145
  stigma and resentment 122
  technology 48

working culture 63, 64–6
working hours 46
working relationships 55, 57
punishment 84–8

redundancy 32, 99
rehabilitation 14, 17, 23, 37, 72
 policy and practice 113, 116, 118
 return to work 33–4
 stigma and resentment 123
repetitive strain injury (RSI) 94, 128
resentment 68, 121–6, 132, 159
 CBT 155, 157
 visibility 128, 130
resignations 31, 32, 99
responsibilization 153, 154, 155, 157, 158, 160
retention of jobs 10, 18, 23
return to work 10, 12–14, 33–5, 118–19
 government policy 14–15
 healthy workplaces 20
 interventions 16, 18
 resentment 125, 160
 staged 74–5
 visibility 126, 128–31

schizo-affective disorder 71
selective serotonin reuptake inhibitors (SSRIs) 3
self-care 154
self-consciousness 69
self-employment 59, 140, 148
self-esteem 60
self-worth 2, 43–4, 58, 60, 67
service sector 11, 16, 34, 135
short-term contracts 65
sick pay 19, 76, 80, 89
sickness absence (sick leave) 13, 32, 34, 65, 71, 108–10
 adjustments 72
 Black Report 22
 healthy workplaces 20–1
 identity 74, 76, 80, 94–5

identity discipline 87–8
identity negotiation 80–2
interventions 17
isolation 67
line managers 101
policy 99, 100
policy and practice 114, 119, 120
productivity obligations 106
resentment 123, 125–6, 155, 160
stress 50, 53, 108, 110
substandard employees 88–92
visibility 127–31
signposting 19
social inclusion 19
social isolation 67, 72, 107, 158
social relations 11, 68, 102–3, 150–1, 159–62
 CBT 154, 155, 156, 158
social skills 17, 33
socio-economics 2, 12, 72
software industry 28
staged returns to work 74–5
stigma 23, 31–3, 37, 85–6, 121–6, 132
 identities 68, 72
 policy 99, 100
stress 3, 5, 14, 33–7, 45, 49–54
 CBT 154, 158
 changing employment landscape 27–9
 duty of care 103
 healthy workplaces 20–1
 interventions 16, 17, 18, 34
 managers 50–1, 53, 108, 110, 112
 policy 100
 service sector 11
 sickness absence 50, 53, 108, 110
 sickness identity 78, 80, 81, 95
 stigma and resentment 124
 visibility 126–7, 129–31
work/life balance 6, 134
working culture 51, 53, 65
working hours 47, 50
working relationships 50, 55, 58

subjection 57, 142, 159
    Gorz 8, 43, 59, 64, 67, 102
subjectivities 30–1, 69–70, 93–5
    CBT 154
    identity discipline 84
    identity negotiation 79
    managers 97–8, 118, 120
    neoliberalism 147, 150–1
    stigma and resentment 123
substandard employees 88–92
support 4, 6, 71–3, 88, 98, 131
    duty of care 105
    line managers 101
    policy 100
    policy and practice 112, 114–16, 119–21
    stigma and resentment 121
    substandard employees 91–2
    working culture 64
    working relationships 57–8

technology 45, 48–9, 63
temporary employment 27, 28, 148
terminating replies 77, 78
trade unions 8, 21, 27, 63, 148
training 23, 33, 119–20, 155
treatment 113, 123

unpaid overtime 28

visibility 126–31, 132
voluntary sector 2, 10, 44, 98, 109–10
    duty of care 104
    goal orientation 60–1
    knowledge of mental health 111–12
    productivity obligations 105
    working hours 46

work ethic 152, 158
work/life balance 6–7, 10, 132, 133–45, 153–4, 160–1
    complimentary perspectives 7–8
    policy and practice 114
    working hours 47, 133–4, 138, 140, 143–5
workfare state 36, 160, 161
working conditions 5, 20–4, 33, 36–7, 43, 81
    government policy 15
    neoliberalism 148, 153
    work/life balance 68, 136, 143
working hours 2–3, 5, 8, 45–7, 107
    anxiety and stress 47, 50
    changing employment landscape 27, 29
    duty of care 104
    neoliberalism 148, 160
    policy and practice 113, 114, 116
    staged returns 74–5
    stigma and resentment 123
    technology 48
    visibility 126
    work/life balance 47, 133–4, 138, 140, 143–5
    working culture 46, 62–3, 65
working relationships 40–1, 43–5, 54–8, 68, 102–3
    anxiety and stress 50, 55, 58
    working culture 63–4, 65
workload 16, 28–9, 33–4, 68, 86, 94–5
    adjustments 73, 74
    policy and practice 113
    productivity obligation 105
    resentment 121–6, 155
    substandard employees 92
    visibility 128
    work/life balance 134, 140